THE BEST EV. BABY NAMES FOR IPSWICH TOWN FANS

*33,000+ Names for Your Baby
That Will Last a Lifetime*

Other books by Dolyttle & Seamore

Dr. Young's Guide to Demotivating Employees
Guide To Selling Your Home
The Best Ever Book of .... Jokes
The Best Ever Guide to Demotivation for ....
The Best Ever Book of Money Saving Tips for ....

To find out more, visit

www.amazon.com

The Best Ever Book of
BABY NAMES
For Ipswich Town Fans

*33,000+ Names for Your Baby
That Will Last a Lifetime*

By Julian St. Claire

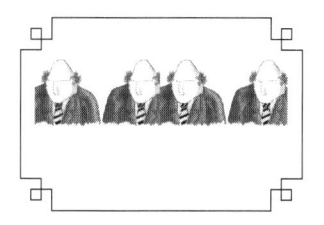

Dolyttle & Seamore
New York, NY

The Best Ever Book of Baby Names: 33,000+ Great Names in a Quick, Easy-To-Use List Format

Dolyttle & Seamore
New York

© Copyright 2014. All rights reserved. No part of this book may be reproduced or transmitted in any form or by any means, electronic or mechanical, including photocopying, recording, digitizing, Web distribution, information storage, distribution and retrieval systems, without the written permission of the publisher.

Limit of Liability/Disclaimer of Warranty: While every effort has been made to ensure the reliability and accuracy of the information contained herein, Dolyttle & Seamore make no representations or warranties with respect to the accuracy or completeness of this book, or the truth of any of the statements. It comes with no warranties, implied or otherwise, of merchantability or fitness for a particular purpose. Neither the publisher or author shall be liable for any damages or losses. This includes, but is not limited to special, incidental, consequential or other damages.

Dolyttle & Seamore
198 Garth Road Suite 2DD
Scarsdale, NY 10583

Publisher's Cataloging-in-Publication Data

The Best Ever Book of Baby Names: 33,000+ Great Names in a Quick, Easy-To-Use List Format

p. cm.
ISBN-13: 9781503056534
ISBN-10:1503056538

10 9 8 7 6 5 4 3 2 1

Julian Syt
Adrea Satre Cover art

Dedicated to my wife, Pam, who could have used this book when our son was born.

Table Of Contents

Introduction ix
Boys Names 11
Girls Names 63

Introduction

Choosing the right name for your child is a difficult and time-consuming process. Parents-to-be obsess about making the right choice, worry about making a mistake after they've made a decision and put too much weight on other people's opinions.

To simplify the process, most parents purchase a baby-naming book. Unfortunately, this often causes confusion and makes an already difficult task even more difficult. Apart from overwhelming them with hundreds, or thousands of pages of useless data, most of these books are filled information that's not needed or wanted.

While parents generally want only one or two names for their child, many put together a list of 50 or 60 names, and whittle it down from there. That means there are tens of thousands of names you're not interested in. Narrowing down this list with most books is time-consuming because you're forced to wade through all of the information about a name, its origins, popularity, age, history, geography, etc.

While you may want this information later for the names you're interested in, you don't need it when you begin your search for the perfect name. This book simplifies the initial process by providing you with an easy-to-follow list that only has names on it.

To use this book:

    1. Highlight the names you like and compile your list.
    2. Edit your list.
    3. Consult your partner.

4. Edit the list again.
5. Continue the process until the list is manageable.

Then, go to the Internet and find out everything you want to know about the names you ACTUALLY like. This will save you a huge amount of time in your quest for the perfect name.

This book has more than 33,000 names in it. Some are obvious, some are unusual, and some are so crazy, you'll wonder how any sane parent-to-be could even consider these names. Rest easy, the purpose of this book is to get you to think outside the box and expand your horizons.

While some of the names may seem strange or unsuitable for Ipswich Town Fans, remember, the purpose of this book is to stimulate your brain and make you consider a variety of different options.

Use this book as your starting point. Change the spelling. Combine names. Use a boy's name on a girl—or vice-versa. It's your child. Don't worry about what other people think. Their advice is worth exactly what you pay for it—nothing.

While you don't need to worry about what other people think, do consider the impact of the name you choose. While almost everything goes in today's enlightened society, naming your son Sue, does still have a few drawbacks!

Good luck in your quest for the perfect name for your child. I hope that this book opens up your eyes to what's possible and helps simplify the process.

Julian St. Claire
Twin Lakes, Wisconsin

Boys Names

A

Aad	Abayomi	Abiel	Achava	Adan	Adken
Aadam	Abba	Abijah	Achelous	Adar	Adkins
Aadan	Abbas	Abilene	Acheron	Adare	Adlai
Aaden	Abbey	Abimael	Achidan	Adarsh	Adler
Aadi	Abbot	Abimelech	Achilles	Adda	Adley
Aadrian	Abbott	Abiola	Achille	Addae	Adli
Aage	Abby	Abir	Achilles	Addai	Admes
Aaidan	Abda	Abiram	Achiram	Addam	Admetus
Aaiden	Abdalah	Abisha	Achishar	Addan	Admon
Aaidyn	Abdalla	Abiyram	Achlys	Addar	Adnah
Aakil	Abdallah	Able	Aciano	Adden	Adnan
Aali	Abdalrahman	Abner	Acim	Addey	Adney
Aalok	Abdel	Abooksigun	Acis	Addis	Adniel
Aalto	Abderus	Abraam	Acker	Addison	Adok
Aapo	Abdi	Abraham	Ackerley	Addo	Adolf
Aarav	Abdiel	Abrahem	Ackley	Addolgar	Adolfo
Aaren	Abdu	Abram	Acoose	Addonis	Adolph
Aaric	Abdukrahman	Abramo	Acotas	Addy	Adolphe
Aaro	Abdul	Abran	Acrisius	Ade	Adolphus
Aaron	Abdulkareem	Abrasha	Actaeon	Adeben	Adom
Aaronn	Abdulla	Abraxas	Acteon	Adeen	Adon
Aarron	Abdullah	Absolom	Acton	Adel	Adonai
Aart	Abdulrahman	Absyrtus	Adael	Adelfuns	Adonia
Aaru	Abe	Abt	Adagio	Adelio	Adonijah
Aarush	Abednago	Abu	Adahy	Adelmar	Adonis
Aatami	Abeeku	Abukcheech	Adaiah	Adelphe	Adonnis
Aatto	Abejundio	Abundio	Adair	Adelphos	Adorellan
Aaydan	Abel	Abush	Adal	Aden	Adras
Aba	Abelard	Abydos	Adalard	Adenn	Adrastos
Abacus	Abelardo	Acacio	Adalbert	Adeon	Adrastus
Aballach	Abell	Acacius	Adalfieri	Aderet	Adresin
Aban	Aberdeen	Academicus	Adalgiso	Adham	Adriaan
Abanito	Aberthol	Acastus	Adalhard	Adhit	Adrian
Abanu	Aberto	Acciai	Adalius	Adi	Adrianno
Abarat	Abhainn	Accius	Adalric	Adib	Adriano
Abarron	Abhay	Ace	Adalrich	Adiba	Adriel
Abasalom	Abi	Acel	Adalwen	Adiel	Adriell
Abasi	Abia	Acelin	Adalwolf	Adil	Adrien
Abay	Abiah	Achaius	Adam	Adin	Adrik
	Abid	Achak	Adamar	Adir	Adrion
	Abida	Achates	Adamm	Aditya	Adriyel
	Abie	Achav	Adamson	Adiv	Adulio

Advent	Aguistin	Aimilios	Akmal	Albee	Aleksy
Adwr	Agung	Aimo	Akon	Alben	Alem
Aeacus	Agustin	Aimon	Akoni	Albern	Aleph
Aed	Agustine	Aindrea	Akos	Albert	Aleron
Aedd	Ahab	Aindreas	Akram	Alberto	Alessandro
Aeetes	Ahanu	Aindriu	Aksel	Albin	Alessio
Aegaeus	Aharon	Ainmire	Akshan	Albinus	Alex
Aegeus	Ahearn	Ainsley	Aktaion	Albion	Alexa
Aegis	Ahearne	Ainslie	Aku	Albondiel	Alexander
Aegisthus	Aherin	Ainsworth	Akub	Albrecht	Alexandras
Aegyptus	Aherne	Aio	Akuji	Albus	Alexandre
Aekerley	Ahiga	Airell	Akule	Alcander	Alexandro
Aelfdane	Ahijah	Airlie	Akuna	Alchemy	Alexandros
Aelrindel	Ahmaad	Aisley	Al	Alcinoos	Alexandrukas
Aeneas	Ahmad	Aitan	Ala	Alcinous	Alexavier
Aenedleah	Ahman	Aithlin	Alaan	Alcnaeon	Alexei
Aenescumb	Ahmed	Aj	Alabama	Alcott	Alexey
Aengus	Ahmik	Aja	Alabaster	Alcyoneus	Alexi
Aeolus	Ahmoua	Ajamu	Alabyran	Aldan	Alexio
Aerendyl	Ahote	Ajani	Aladdin	Alddes	Alexios
Aesculapius	Ahren	Ajax	Alagan	Alden	Alexis
Aesir	Ahsalom	Ajay	Alai	Alder	Alexius
Aeson	Ahsan	Akalanka	Alain	Aldin	Alexxander
Aesop	Ahtunowhiho	Akamu	Alair	Aldis	Alexzander
Aethelberht	Aiattaua	Akando	Alaire	Aldo	Alf
Aethelbert	Aibhne	Akay	Alamar	Aldon	Alfarin
Aetos	Aibne	Akbar	Alamo	Aldous	Alfie
Afal	Aidan	Ake	Alan	Aldred	Alfio
Afamrail	Aidann	Akecheta	Alani	Aldric	Alfonso
Afif	Aiddan	Akeem	Alann	Aldrich	Alford
Afton	Aidden	Akello	Alano	Aldrick	Alfred
Agamedes	Aiden	Akeno	Alanzo	Aldrin	Alfredo
Agamemnon	Aidenn	Akhenaten	Alaois	Aldwin	Alfrothul
Agape	Aidrian	Aki	Alard	Aldwine	Algar
Agapito	Aidric	Akia	Alaric	Alec	Alger
Agassi	Aidyn	Akiba	Alarick	Aleck	Algernon
Agastya	Aiiden	Akihiko	Alarico	Aled	Algie
Agathias	Aiken	Akihito	Alarik	Aleem	Algis
Agatone	Ail	Akikta	Alary	Alef	Algot
Ager	Ailbert	Akil	Alasd	Alejandro	Algrenon
Aghaderg	Ailean	Akim	Alasdair	Alejo	Alhan
Aghamore	Ailein	Akins	Alastair	Alek	Ali
Aghy	Ailesh	Akintunde	Alaula	Alekanekelo	Alian
Agilan	Ailfrid	Akio	Alawi	Aleko	Aliceson
Agis	Ailill	Akir	Alawn	Aleksandar	Alick
Agni	Ailin	Akira	Alba	Aleksander	Alii
Agnolo	Aillig	Akiro	Alban	Aleksandr	Alijah
Agostino	Aim	Akito	Albanwr	Aleksei	Alik
Agrican	Aime	Akiva	Albany	Aleksi	Alim
Agu	Aimery	Akkar	Albaric	Aleksis	Alimayu

12

Alinar	Alrik	Amarey	Amin	Amzi	Andrea
Alis	Alroy	Amari	Aminadav	An	Andreas
Alison	Alson	Amarillo	Amir	Anacletus	Andrei
Alistair	Alston	Amarion	Amiram	Anacreon	Andren
Alistaire	Alta	Amasa	Amiri	Anael	Andreo
Alister	Altaf	Amasai	Amirr	Anakausuen	Andres
Alivia	Altair	Amathaon	Amis	Anakin	Andreus
Alix	Altan	Amato	Amish	Anakoni	Andrew
Allan	Alter	Amatzya	Amisquew	Analu	Andrey
Allard	Althidon	Amaud	Amit	Ananda	Andrian
Allaster	Altman	Amaury	Amita	Anando	Andriel
Allec	Alto	Amaziah	Amitai	Anane	Andries
Allen	Alton	Amazu	Amiti	Anang	Andrik
Allexander	Alucio	Ambar	Amjad	Anarawd	Andrin
Allie	Aluf	Ambrocio	Amlawdd	Anas	Andrion
Allijah	Aluin	Ambrogio	Amma	Anasazi	Androcles
Allison	Aluino	Ambroise	Amman	Anass	Androgeus
Allister	Alun	Ambrose	Ammar	Anastagio	Androu
Allonzo	Alured	Ambrosi	Ammi	Anastasio	Andrusha
Ally	Alva	Ambrosio	Ammiel	Anastasios	Andrya
Almanzo	Alvah	Ambrus	Ammiras	Anastasius	Andwele
Almarine	Alvan	Amd	Ammitai	Anasztaz	Andy
Almas	Alvar	Ame	Ammon	Anatol	Aneirin
Almonzo	Alvaro	Amedeo	Amnchadh	Anatole	Aneislis
Alo	Alvern	Amedeus	Amnon	Anatoli	Aneurin
Aloeus	Alvin	Ameer	Amo	Anatolii	Anfalen
Aloha	Alvino	Amell	Amoldo	Anatolijus	Anfernee
Alohilani	Alvis	Amen	Amon	Anatolio	Anfri
Aloiki	Alwin	Amenhotep	Amor	Anatoliy	Ang
Aloin	Alwyn	Amerawdwr	Amory	Anaximander	Angaros
Alok	Aly	Amergin	Amos	Anbessa	Angawdd
Alon	Alyosha	America	Amot	Ancaeus	Angel
Alonso	Amaari	Americus	Amotz	Ancelin	Angelico
Alonzo	Amad	Amerigo	Amou	Anchises	Angelino
Alosrin	Amadeo	Amery	Amour	Anchor	Angelito
Aloyoshenka	Amadeus	Ames	Amoux	Ancil	Angell
Aloysha	Amadi	Amethyst	Amphiaraus	Anddy	Angello
Aloysius	Amado	Ameya	Amphion	Ande	Angelo
Alp	Amadour	Amhar	Amphitryon	Andenon	Anghrist
Alperen	Amael	Amhlaoibh	Ampyx	Ander	Angor
Alpha	Amahl	Amhuinn	Amram	Anders	Angus
Alpheus	Amal	Ami	Amren	Anderson	Anibal
Alphonse	Amalio	Amiad	Amrit	Andersson	Anicho
Alphonso	Aman	Amias	Amrynn	Andie	Anik
Alphonsus	Amancio	Amichai	Amsterdam	Andino	Aniketos
Alpin	Amaoebus	Amid	Amsu	Andnej	Aniol
Alpine	Amar	Amiel	Amyas	Andor	Anlon
Alric	Amaram	Amiir	Amycus	Andras	Anlyth
Alrick	Amaranth	Amikam	Amynedd	Andrathath	Annan
Alrigo	Amare	Amil	Amyneddgar	Andre	Anndy

13

Anoki	Anwir	Arata	Argo	Arley	Arrio
Anscom	Anwyl	Arathorn	Argos	Arlin	Arron
Anse	Anwyll	Aratus	Argus	Arliss	Arrow
Ansel	Anynnawg	Arav	Argyle	Arlo	Arroyo
Ansell	Anyon	Arawn	Ari	Arman	Arsen
Anselm	Anzel	Arbane	Ariabod	Armand	Arsenio
Anselmo	Aodh	Arber	Arian	Armande	Arsenios
Ansgar	Aodhan	Arbor	Aribert	Armandek	Art
Anshel	Aoi	Arcadicus	Aric	Armando	Artair
Anshu	Aoibheann	Arcadio	Arich	Armani	Artan
Ansley	Aoidh	Arcas	Aricin	Armann	Artaxiad
Anson	Aoki	Arcelio	Arick	Armanno	Artegal
Anstice	Aolani	Arcenio	Arie	Armen	Artem
Anstiss	Aolis	Arch	Ariel	Armin	Artemas
Antaeus	Aonghas	Archaimbaud	Arien	Armistead	Artemesio
Antanas	Aonghus	Archambault	Aries	Armo	Artemii
Antares	Apenimon	Archard	Arif	Armon	Artemis
Antenor	Aphrodite	Archelaus	Arik	Armond	Artemus
Anteros	Apiatan	Archemorus	Arion	Armondo	Arthel
Anthonny	Apollinaire	Archenhaud	Aris	Armstrong	Arthgallo
Anthony	Apollo	Archer	Aristaeus	Arnaldo	Arthur
Antilochus	Apollodorus	Archibald	Aristedes	Arnan	Arthwr
Antinko	Apollos	Archibaldo	Aristeo	Arnat	Artie
Antinous	Apolonio	Archie	Aristides	Arnatt	Artis
Antioco	Apoloniusz	Archimedes	Aristo	Arnau	Artois
Antionne	Aponivi	Archwood	Aristos	Arnaud	Artur
Antiphates	Apostol	Ardagh	Aristotle	Arnav	Arturo
Antoine	Apostolos	Ardal	Arius	Arne	Artus
Antoinne	Apsel	Ardell	Arizona	Arnet	Arty
Anton	Apu	Arden	Arjan	Arnett	Arun
Antonin	Aqil	Ardghal	Arjay	Arni	Aruna
Antonino	Aquarius	Ardian	Arjen	Arnie	Arundel
Antonio	Aquila	Ardin	Arjun	Arno	Arvad
Antonius	Aquilan	Ardkill	Arjuna	Arnold	Arval
Antonnio	Aquilino	Ardley	Arkadi	Arnoldo	Arve
Antonny	Aquilo	Ardmore	Arkadios	Arnon	Arvel
Antony	Aquinnah	Ardolf	Arkadiy	Arnulf	Arvid
Antoon	Aquino	Ardolph	Arkady	Arnulfo	Arvil
Antor	Ara	Ardon	Arkansas	Aroghetto	Arvin
Antosha	Arabia	Ardreth	Arkasha	Aron	Arvind
Antranig	Araby	Ardryll	Arketah	Aroon	Arwan
Antwan	Aragon	Arduino	Arkhippos	Aros	Arwel
Anubis	Aragorn	Ardwyad	Arkin	Arpad	Ary
Anund	Aralt	Areli	Arkyn	Arran	Aryaan
Anwar	Aram	Aren	Arl	Arregaithel	Aryan
Anwas	Aramis	Arend	Arlan	Arri	Aryasb
Anwell	Aran	Ares	Arland	Arrian	Arye
Anwer	Aranck	Argent	Arlando	Arric	Aryeh
Anwil	Araris	Argento	Arledge	Arrick	Asa
Anwill	Arash	Arglwydd	Arlen	Arrigo	Asad

Asael	Aston	Aubrey	Author	Avshalom	Azim
Asaf	Astraeus	Aubron	Autolycus	Awan	Aziz
Asahavey	Astro	Aubry	Autry	Aweinon	Aziza
Asahel	Aswin	Auburn	Ava	Awendea	Azize
Asahi	Ata	Auckland	Avak	Awendela	Azizi
Asaiah	Atahladte	Audel	Avallach	Awinita	Azra
Asante	Atahualpa	Auden	Avalon	Awnan	Azrael
Asaph	Atallah	Audey	Avaon	Awstin	Azrie
Asbjørn	Atalo	Audi	Avarair	Axeel	Azriel
Ascal	Ataullah	Audie	Avatar	Axel	Azul
Ascalaphus	Atemu	Audio	Avdel	Axell	Azure
Ascanius	Athamas	Audley	Avedis	Axl	Azzam
Ascot	Athan	Audric	Avel	Axton	Azzedine
Asen	Athanasios	Audrick	Avenall	Axxel	
Asgard	Athanasius	Audwin	Aveneil	Ayaan	**B**
Asgrim	Athdar	August	Avenelle	Ayaki	
Ash	Athelstan	Augusten	Avent	Ayal	Baba
Ashanti	Athemar	Augustin	Averett	Ayarn	Baback
Ashbel	Athens	Augustine	Averil	Ayawamat	Babak
Ashburn	Atherton	Augusto	Averill	Aydan	Babson
Ashby	Athol	Augustus	Avernus	Aydann	Babu
Ashe	Athos	Augusty	Avery	Aydden	Baby
Asher	Athtar	Augustyn	Avi	Aydeen	Bac
Ashes	Athumani	Auhert	Aviad	Ayden	Baccaus
Ashford	Atif	Aulani	Avichai	Aydin	Bacchus
Ashkan	Atish	Auley	Avidan	Ayele	Baccus
Ashkii	Atius	Aulii	Avidor	Ayers	Bach
Ashland	Atkins	Aumanas	Aviel	Ayinde	Bachelor
Ashley	Atl	Aumrauth	Avigdor	Aylmer	Badan
Asho	Atlas	Aure	Avignon	Aylward	Badar
Ashok	Atle	Aurek	Avihu	Aylwin	Badden
Ashraf	Atlee	Aureli	Avimelech	Ayman	Baddon
Ashton	Atley	Aurelian	Avinadav	Ayu	Bade
Ashur	Atli	Aureliano	Avinoam	Ayunli	Baden
Ashwin	Atreo	Aurélien	Aviram	Ayzize	Bader
Asif	Atreus	Aurelio	Avis	Az	Badr
Asim	Atsushi	Aurelius	Avish	Aza	Badrick
Ask	Atticus	Auren	Avisha	Azaiah	Badru
Askel	Attie	Auric	Avishai	Azam	Baeddan
Asklepios	Attila	Aurick	Avital	Azaria	Baen
Askook	Attis	Aurik	Aviv	Azariah	Baer
Aslan	Atu	Auriville	Avner	Azarias	Baez
Asmara	Atuf	Aurum	Avniel	Azarious	Baggio
Asmund	Atum	Ausar	Avon	Azaryah	Baha
Asopus	Atwater	Austen	Avonaco	Azaryahu	Bahadur
Aspen	Atwell	Auster	Avourel	Azel	Baham
Assan	Atwood	Austin	Avraham	Azhar	Bahari
Assar	Atworth	Austinn	Avram	Azia	Bahram
Asthore	Auberon	Austyn	Avrum	Azibo	Baigh
Astin	Aubin	Autha	Avsalom	Aziel	Bail

15

Bailey	Banan	Barker	Barzillai	Beacon	Bekele
Balloch	Banbhan	Barksdale	Bas	Beagan	Bel
Bain	Bancroft	Barley	Base	Beal	Bela
Bainbridge	Bandana	Barlow	Bash	Beale	Belanor
Bairam	Bandele	Barn	Basie	Beall	Belay
Baird	Bandit	Barnab	Basil	Beaman	Belcher
Bairn	Bane	Barnabas	Basile	Beamard	Beldane
Bakari	Bangkok	Barnabe	Basilio	Beamer	Belden
Baker	Bani	Barnaby	Basim	Bean	Beldene
Baki	Banji	Barnard	Basir	Bear	Beldroth
Baku	Banjo	Barnardo	Baskara	Bearach	Belen
Bala	Banks	Barnes	Bassett	Bearchán	BeliMawr
Balagtas	Banner	Barneston	Bast	Bearnard	Belindo
Balasi	Banning	Barnett	Baste	Beartlaidh	Belisario
Balbo	Bannock	Barney	Bastet	Beasley	Bell
Baldasarre	Bansi	Barnum	Bastiaan	Beathan	Bellamy
Baldassario	Banyan	Barny	Bastian	Beattie	Bellarmine
Baldemar	Banys	Baron	Bastien	Beatty	Bellas
Balder	Bao	Barr	Bastijn	Beau	Bellerophon
Baldhere	Baptist	Barrak	Bat	Beauchamp	Bello
Baldie	Baptiste	Barram	Batair	Beaufort	Bellow
Baldr	Baqer	Barras	Bates	Beaumont	Belmont
Baldric	Baqir	Barrett	Bathsheba	Beauregard	Belton
Baldur	Barabas	Barric	Batson	Beauvais	Beltran
Baldwin	Barabbas	Barrie	Battista	Beaver	Beluar
Bale	Barack	Barrin	Batu	Becan	Belvedere
Balen	Barak	Barrington	Batul	Becher	Bem
Balfour	Barakat	Barris	Batzorig	Bechet	Bemabe
Balgair	Baram	Barron	Baucis	Beck	Bembe
Balgaire	Baraz	Barry	Bauer	Becker	Bemossed
Bali	Barbeau	Bart	Baxley	Beckett	Bemus
Balin	Barber	Barta	Baxter	Beckham	Ben
Balint	Barbod	Bartel	Bay	Beda	Benaiah
Ballard	Barbossa	Barth	Bayanai	Bede	Benard
Balliol	Barclay	Bartholemew	Bayard	Bedell	Benat
Ballou	Bard	Bartholomew	Bayle	Bedros	Benci
Balmoral	Bardan	Bartleby	Baylee	Bedwyr	Bendek
Balsam	Barday	Bartlet	Baylen	Bedyw	Bendigeidfran
Baltasar	Barden	Bartlett	Bayless	Beech	Bendyk
Balthasar	Bardene	Bartley	Bayley	Beecher	Benecroft
Balthazar	Bardia	Barto	Bayou	Behan	Benedetto
Baltimore	Bardo	Bartol	Bayron	Behar	Benedick
Balton	Bardolf	Bartoli	Bayu	Behdad	Benedict
Baltsaros	Bardolph	Bartolo	Baz	Behitha	Benedicto
Balzac	Bardot	Bartolome	Baze	Behnam	Benedictson
Bama	Bardrick	Barton	Bazel	Behruz	Benen
Bamboo	Barek	Bartram	Bazyli	Beige	Benevolent
Ban	Barend	Bartt	Beacan	Beinvenido	Beniamino
Banagher	Barid	Baruch	Beach	Beirne	Benicio
Banaing	Barke	Bary	Beacher	Beiste	Benigno

Benin	Berkeley	Bhradain	Birr	Blue	Borka
Benito	Berkley	Bhraghad	Birtle	Bly	Borna
Benjamen	Berlin	Bhreac	Birungi	Bo	Borromeo
Benjamin	Berlyn	Bhric	Bishop	Boas	Borya
Benjammin	Bern	Biafyndar	Biton	Boaz	Boryenka
Benjen	Bernado	Biaggio	Bix	Bob	Borys
Benji	Bernal	Biagio	Bjergen	Bobby	Boryslaw
Benjiro	Bernard	Biaiardo	Bjorn	Bodaway	Bosco
Benjy	Bernardo	Bialaer	Bjornson	Bode	Bosley
Benkamin	Bernardyn	Bialas	Black	Boden	Boston
Benn	Berne	Bialy	Blackburn	Bodhi	Boswell
Bennet	Bernelle	Biast	Blackburne	Bodi	Bosworth
Bennett	Bernhard	Bickford	Blackstone	Bodie	Botan
Bennie	Bernie	Bid	Blackwell	Bogart	Bothain
Benning	Bernon	Bidaban	Blade	Bogdan	Botham
Benniton	Bernt	Bidziil	Blagden	Bogdashha	Bothan
Bennjamin	Berny	Bien	Blain	Bogomil	Botolf
Benno	Berold	Bienne	Blaine	Bogumil	Boudewijn
Benny	Berquist	Bienvenido	Blair	Boguslaw	Bourbon
Beno	Berry	Biff	Blais	Bohan	Bourne
Benoit	Bert	Bige	Blaisdell	Bohdan	Boutros
Benoni	Berta	Bijan	Blaise	Bohemond	Bouvier
Benroy	Berth	Bijou	Blaize	Boinedal	Bowen
Benson	Berthold	Bijoux	Blake	Bolan	Bowie
Bente	Berti	Bilagaana	Blakeley	Bolivar	Boy
Bentlee	Bertie	Bilal	Blakely	Bolivia	Boyce
Bentley	Bertin	Bill	Blakeney	Bolodenka	Boyd
Bently	Berto	Billie	Blanco	Bolton	Boyden
Benton	Berton	Billy	Blandino	Boman	Boyer
Benvenuto	Bertram	Bima	Blane	Bombay	Boyko
Benvolio	Bertrand	Bimini	Blaney	Bonamy	Boyne
Benyamin	Bertrando	Bimisi	Blanford	Bonanza	Boynton
Benzion	Berwin	Bimo	Blanket	Bonar	Boys
Beolagh	Berwyn	Bin	Blanton	Bonaventure	Bozrah
Beowulf	Beryl	Binah	Blaque	Bond	Brac
Berakhiah	Betelgeuse	Binda	Blar	Boniface	Bracken
Bered	Bethel	Binder	Blas	Bonifacio	Brad
Berenger	Betzalel	Bing	Blase	Bonifaco	Bradaigh
Beres	Beval	Bingham	Blathaon	Bonifacy	Bradan
Beresford	Bevan	Bingo	Blathma	Bonner	Bradburn
Berg	Beven	Binh	Blayne	Bono	Bradbury
Bergan	Beverly	Binky	Blayze	Boo	Bradd
Bergar	Bevin	Binyamin	Blaze	Booker	Bradden
Berger	Bevis	Birch	Bleddyn	Boone	Braddock
Berggren	Bevyn	Birchall	Bleicher	Booth	Braddon
Beriah	Beynon	Bird	Bleidd	Borak	Braden
Berilo	Bezai	Birkett	Blian	Borden	Bradey
Berin	Bhaic	Birkey	Bligh	Boreas	Bradford
Berinhard	Bhaltair	Birley	Bliss	Borg	Bradlee
Berke	Bhavya	Birney	Blondell	Boris	Bradley

Bradly	Brant	Brendan	Brinkley	Brunelle	Burian
Bradman	Brantlee	Brenden	Brinley	Bruno	Burke
Bradon	Brantley	Brendon	Brinly	Brutus	Burl
Bradshaw	Brantly	Brends	Brinsley	Bryan	Burleigh
Bradwen	Branton	Brendyn	Brinton	Bryant	Burley
Bradwr	Brantson	Brenen	Brio	Bryce	Burma
Brady	Branxton	Brenn	Brishan	Brycen	Burnaby
Bradyn	Braoin	Brennan	Bristol	Bryden	Burne
Braedan	Braque	Brenndan	Brit	Brydon	Burnet
Braeden	Brasen	Brennden	Britain	Brygus	Burnett
Braedon	Brasidas	Brenndon	Britt	Bryn	Burney
Braedyn	Brasil	Brennen	Britton	Bryne	Burns
Braen	Brason	Brenner	Broc	Brynn	Burr
Braern	Brathach	Brennon	Brochan	Brynner	Burris
Braham	Braulio	Brent	Brock	Bryon	Burroughs
Brahms	Braun	Brenten	Brockton	Brys	Burt
Braiden	Bravery	Brentley	Brocky	Brysen	Burton
Braidon	Bravo	Brently	Brod	Bryson	Busby
Braima	Brawley	Brenton	Brodderick	Brysonn	Busch
Brain	Braxon	Brentt	Broden	Bryston	Buster
Brainard	Braxton	Brentton	Broder	Bryton	Butades
Braison	Braxxton	Breslin	Broderic	Buana	Butch
Bram	Bray	Bret	Broderick	Bubba	Butcher
Bramwell	Brayan	Breton	Brodie	Buchanan	Butler
Bran	Brayden	Brett	Brodny	Buck	Button
Branagan	Braydenn	Bretton	Brodric	Buckley	Buzz
Branch	Braydon	Brevin	Brodrick	Buckminster	Bwlch
Brand	Braylen	Brevyn	Brody	Bud	Byatt
Brandan	Braylon	Brewster	Broehain	Buddy	Byford
Branddon	Brayton	Breyon	Brogan	Buell	Byme
Brandeis	Braz	Breyson	Brom	Buenaventura	Byram
Branden	Brazier	Brian	Bromley	Buff	Byran
Brandenn	Brazil	Briar	Bron	Buford	Byrd
Brander	Breac	Briareus	Bronco	Buinton	Byrne
Brandin	Breaker	Brice	Brone	Buiron	Byron
Brando	Breandan	Bricen	Bronislaw	Bulana	
Brandon	Breasal	Brick	Bronson	Bull	

C

Brandonn	Breccan	Bricriu	Bronx	Bundy	
Brandt	Breck	Bridge	Brook	Bunta	Caaden
Brandyn	Brecken	Bridger	Brooke	Bunyan	Cab
Branigan	Breckin	Brier	Brooklee	Burbank	Caballero
Branislav	Breckinridge	Brieuc	Brooklyn	Burcet	Cabe
Branko	Brede	Briggs	Brooks	Burch	Cable
Branley	Breed	Brigham	Broox	Burdan	Cabot
Brannan	Breen	Brighton	Brosh	Burdett	Cacanisius
Branndon	Breindel	Brilane	Brosnan	Burdette	Cace
Brannen	Bremen	Brileigh	Brown	Burel	Cacey
Brannon	Bren	Briley	Bruce	Burford	Cache
Bransen	Brencis	Brilliant	Bruin	Burgess	Cactus
Branson	Brend	Brink	Bruis	Burgundy	Cadao

Cadarn	Caird	Calvagh	Canyon	Carnig	Cassidy
Cadawg	Cairn	Calvert	Caolaidhe	Caro	Cassiel
Cadby	Cairo	Calvin	Caolan	Carol	Cassio
Cadden	Cais	Calvino	Capaneus	Carollan	Cassius
Caddis	Caiseal	Caly	Capp	Carolos	Cassivellaunus
Caddoc	Caith	Calypso	Capri	Carolus	Casson
Caddock	Caius	Cam	Capricorn	Caron	Casswallawn
Cade	Cajetan	Camara	Car	Carpenter	Casta
Cadel	Cal	Camaxtli	Caractacus	Carpus	Castel
Cadell	Caladh	Camber	Caradawg	Carr	Caster
Cadellin	Calais	Cambeul	Caradoc	Carraig	Castiel
Caden	Calan	Camdan	Caradog	Carrick	Castor
Cadence	Calbert	Camden	Caraidland	Carrigan	Caswallon
Cadfael	Calbhach	Camdin	Carbry	Carrington	Catahecassa
Cadfan	Calcas	Camdyn	Cardell	Carrol	Cater
Cadman	Calchas	Camedyr	Carden	Carroll	Cath
Cadmon	Calder	Cameo	Carel	Carrson	Cathal
Cadmus	Caldwell	Cameron	Carew	Cars	Cathan
Cadoc	Cale	Camerron	Carey	Carsen	Catlin
Cadogan	Caleb	Camhlaidh	Cargan	Carson	Cato
Caduceus	Caledon	Camilo	Cariad	Carsten	Catullus
Cadwallen	Caledvwlch	Cammeron	Carl	Carswell	Cavalier
Cadwgawn	Calen	Cammron	Carlen	Carsyn	Cavan
Cadwr	Calendar	Camp	Carleton	Carter	Cavanagh
Cadwy	Calev	Campbell	Carley	Carthach	Cavanaugh
Cadyryeith	Caley	Campion	Carlin	Carthage	Cawley
Cael	Calgary	Camren	Carling	Cartland	Cawrdav
Caelan	Calhoun	Camron	Carlino	Caruso	Caxton
Caeo	Caliban	Camryn	Carlisle	Carvell	Cayden
Caerau	Calico	Camshron	Carlo	Carver	Caydenn
Caerleon	California	Can	Carlomagno	Carwyn	Cayman
CaerLlion	Calisto	Canaan	Carlos	Cary	Cayo
Caerwyn	Calix	Canan	Carloss	Cas	Cayson
Caesar	Calixto	Canarsie	Carlow	Case	Caz
Caesare	Callaghan	Canby	Carlsen	Caseareo	Ceallach
Cage	Callahan	Candelario	Carlton	Casen	Cearbhall
Cager	Callan	Candid	Carlus	Casey	Cearbhallan
Cagney	Callaway	Candide	Carly	Cash	Ceard
Cahir	Callen	Candido	Carlyle	Cashel	Ceardach
Cahya	Callias	Candra	Carman	Cashmere	Cearnach
Cai	Callis	Canc	Carmel	Casimir	Cecil
Caiden	Callister	Canfield	Carmelo	Casimiro	Cecilio
Cailean	Callough	Canice	Carmen	Casnar	Cecrops
Cailen	Calloway	Cannan	Carmi	Cason	Cedar
Cailin	Callum	Canning	Carmichael	Caspar	Cederic
Caillen	Calm	Cannon	Carmiel	Casper	Cedric
Cain	Calogero	Canon	Carmine	Caspian	Cedrick
Caine	Calton	Cant	Carne	Cass	Cedrik
Caio	Calum	Canton	Carnell	Cassander	Cedro
Cairbre	Calumet	Canute	Carney	Cassian	Ceithin

Celadon	Chalil	Charis	Chelsea	Chimalus	Churchill
Celestine	Chalkley	Charles	Chelsey	Chimelu	Cian
Celestino	Chalmar	Charleston	Chen	Chinelo	Cianan
Celesto	Chalmer	Charley	Cheney	Chino	Ciar
Celeus	Chalmers	Charlie	Cheng	Chinua	Ciaran
Celio	Chaman	Charlles	Chepe	Chip	Ciarrai
Cellini	Chamberlain	Charlot	Cherokee	Chipper	Cibor
Cello	Chamonix	Charlton	Cherut	Chiram	Cicero
Celso	Champion	Charly	Cheslav	Chirico	Ciceron
Celtic	Chan	Charnell	Chesley	Chisholm	Cid
Celyn	Chanan	Charon	Chesmu	Chitt	Cidro
Cenon	Chananya	Charro	Chesney	Chlyses	Cielo
Cephalus	Chance	Chars	Chester	Chizkiel	Cillian
Cephas	Chancellor	Charsian	Cheston	Chochmo	Cimarron
Cepheus	Chancelor	Charybdis	Chet	Chochokpi	Cimon
Cerbelus	Chand	Chas	Chetan	Chogan	Cincinnatus
Ceres	Chandler	Chaschunka	Chetanluta	Choncey	Cinco
Ceri	Chandra	Chase	Chetanzi	Choni	Cinna
Ceron	Chane	Chasen	Chett	Choovio	Cinneide
Cerulean	Chaney	Chasin	Chetwin	Chovav	Cinnfhail
Cesar	Chang	Chaska	Cheval	Choviohoya	Cionaodh
Cesare	Change	Chasse	Chevalier	Chowilawu	Cipriano
Cesario	Chaniel	Chathanglas	Chevell	Chris	Ciqala
Cesaro	Chanina	Chato	Cheveyo	Christan	Ciriaco
Cetus	Chanler	Chattan	Chevis	Christiaan	Cirilo
Ceylon	Chanlyeya	Chatura	Chevron	Christian	Cirio
Ceyx	Channce	Chaucer	Chevy	Christiano	Ciro
Cha'tima	Channe	Chaunce	Cheyenne	Christiansen	Cirocco
Chace	Channer	Chaunceler	Cheyne	Christianus	Cirrus
Chachi	Channing	Chauncey	Cheyrth	Christie	Cisco
Chad	Channon	Chauncory	Chi	Christien	Citra
Chadbyrne	Chano	Chauncy	Chiamaka	Christmas	Citro
Chadd	Chanoch	Chavakuk	Chiazam	Christo	Clyde
Chaddrick	Chant	Chavez	Chibale	Christoffer	Clywd
Chadrick	Chanter	Chaviv	Chicago	Christofor	Claas
Chadwick	Chantesuta	Chavivi	Chicha	Christoopher	Clach
Chadwik	Chanteyukan	Chay	Chick	Christoph	Claes
Chadwyk	Chantrey	Chayan	Chico	Christophe	Claiborne
Chael	Chantry	Chayim	Chidi	Christopher	Clancy
Chagai	Chao	Chayne	Chikafusa	Christophor	Clarence
Chaggai	Chaos	Chayo	Chikao	Christophoros	Clarion
Chai	Chaparral	Chayton	Chike	Christos	Clark
Chaika	Chapin	Chaz	Chikezie	Christy	Clarke
Chaim	Chaplin	Chazaiah	Chiko	Chruse	Clarrie
Chainey	Chapman	Chazon	Chileab	Chrysostom	Claude
Chairo	Chappel	Chazz	Chili	Chuchip	Claudio
Chait	Chappell	Che	Chilion	Chuck	Claudios
Chakotay	Charaka	Cheche	Chill	Chung	Claudius
Chakra	Charan	Cheever	Chilli	Chunta	Claus
Chalice	Chardon	Chelan	Chilton	Chuong	Claxton

Clay	Clunainach	Coleridge	Conchobhar	Corcoran	Cosmin
Clayborne	Cluny	Coley	Concord	Cord	Cosmo
Clayland	Clust	Colgate	Coney	Cordaro	Costa
Clayne	Cluym	Coligny	Cong	Cordell	Costas
Clayton	Clyde	Colin	Congo	Cordero	Costello
Cleander	Cnut	Coll	Conlan	Corderro	Coster
Cleanth	Cnute	Colla	Conleth	Cordovan	Cotton
Cleary	Cnychwr	Collen	Conley	Corentin	Cottus
Cleatus	Coady	Colley	Conn	Corentine	Coty
Cleavant	Coakley	Collier	Connacht	Corey	Cougar
Cleave	Coal	Collin	Connak	Cori	Coulson
Cleavon	Cobalt	Collins	Connal	Coriander	Coulter
Cledwyn	Cobb	Colm	Connecticut	Coridan	Council
Cleit	Cobden	Colman	Connell	Corin	Count
Clem	Cobham	Colombe	Connelly	Cork	Countee
Clemency	Cobhan	Colony	Conner	Corky	Court
Clemens	Coburn	Colorado	Connery	Corliss	Courtenay
Clement	Coby	Colquhoun	Connie	Cormac	Courtland
Clemente	Coch	Colson	Connla	Cormack	Courtnay
Clennan	Cochise	Colston	Connley	Cormic	Courtney
Cleobis	Cochlain	Colt	Connolly	Cormick	Cove
Cleon	Cockrell	Coltan	Connor	Cornaith	Covell
Cleophas	Cocoa	Colten	Conny	Cornel	Covert
Clete	Cocytus	Colter	Conor	Cornelio	Covey
Cletus	Coddy	Coltin	Conrad	Cornelious	Covington
Cleve	Codell	Colton	Conrado	Cornelius	Covy
Cleveland	Codey	Coltrane	Conran	Cornell	Cowal
Clever	Codie	Coltyn	Constant	Cornellius	Cowan
Cleytus	Cody	Colum	Constantijn	Cornwallis	Cowrie
Cliff	Coe	Columba	Constantin	Coro	Cox
Clifford	Coed	Columbo	Constantine	Corradeo	Coy
Cliffton	Coen	Columbus	Constantino	Corrado	Coyan
Clifland	Coeur	Colville	Consuel	Corran	Coye
Clifton	Coeus	Colwyn	Conway	Corren	Coyle
Clint	Coffin	Colyn	Cony	Correy	Coyne
Clinton	Cohen	Coman	Conyers	Corridon	Coyotl
Clio	Cohnal	Comanche	Conyn	Corrin	Coz
Clitus	Coilin	Comfort	Cook	Cort	Craddock
Clive	Coillcumhann	Comhghall	Cookie	Cortez	Cradoe
Clodoveo	Coinneach	Comhghan	Coolio	Cortland	Craig
Clooney	Coire	Como	Cooper	Corvin	Cramer
Clotilde	Coireall	Comstock	Cope	Corwin	Crandall
Cloud	Colan	Comus	Corban	Cory	Crane
Clourindo	Colbert	Comyn	Corbeau	Corybantes	Cranford
Clove	Colbey	Con	Corben	Corydon	Cranley
Cloven	Colburn	Conaire	Corbett	Corym	Crannog
Clovis	Colby	Conal	Corbin	Cos	Cranston
Cloy	Colden	Conall	Corbinian	Cosgrove	Crash
Clud	Cole	Conan	Corby	Cosimo	Craven
Cluhurach	Coleman	Conary	Corbyn	Cosmas	Crawford

21

Cray	Croydon	Cy	Dagobert	Dalyor	Danil
Crayton	Cru	Cyan	Dagon	Dalziel	Danila
Cree	Cruadhlaoich	Cycnus	Dagwood	Damae	Danilo
Creed	Crue	Cyd	Dahl	Damalis	Danish
Creedon	Cruim	Cydney	Dahy	Daman	Dann
Creek	Crusoe	Cymbeline	Dai	Damani	Dannel
Creighton	Cruz	Cymry	Daibheid	Damarcus	Danner
Creola	Cruzito	Cynbal	Daichi	Damario	Dannie
Creon	Csaba	Cynbel	Daijiro	Damarion	Danniell
Crescent	Csongor	Cyneley	Daiki	Damaris	Danno
Crespin	Ctesippus	Cyprian	Daileass	Damaskenos	Dannon
Cresswell	Cualli	Cyprus	Dailey	Damaskinos	Danny
Cretien	Cuanaic	Cyr	Daimh	Damaso	Dano
Crevan	Cuartio	Cyrano	Daimhin	Damek	Dantae
Crew	Cuarto	Cyrek	Dain	Damen	Dante
Crichton	Cuba	Cyril	Dainard	Dameon	Dantee
Cricket	Cubert	Cyrille	Daine	Damian	Dantel
Crimson	Cuinn	Cyrus	Daire	Damiann	Danton
Criostoir	Culhwch	Cyryl	Daishiro	Damiano	Dantrell
Cris	Cullen	Cystennin	Daisuke	Damien	Danube
Crisanto	Culley	Czar	Daitaro	Damion	Danya
Crispin	Cullinan	Czeslaw	Daithi	Damir	Danyal
Crispus	Cullo		Daivat	Dammian	Danyl
Crist	Culloden	**D**	Dajon	Dammon	Danylko
Cristian	Culvanawd		Dajuan	Damocles	Daoud
Cristiano	Culver	D'anton	Dakarai	Damon	Daphnis
Cristobal	Cumhea	D'Arcy	Dakath	Damond	Daquan
Cristofer	Cunnawabum	D'arcy	Dakila	Damonn	Dar
Cristofor	Cunningham	D'Artagnan	Dakoda	Damyan	Dara
Cristoforo	Cupid	Daan	Dakota	Dan	Darach
Criston	Curcio	Dabi	Dakotah	Dana	Daray
Cristophe	Curley	Dabney	Dal	Danail	Darby
Cristopher	Curragh	Dace	Dalan	Danar	Darcassan
Cristos	Curran	Dacey	Dalbert	Danaus	Darcel
Cristoval	Currier	Dacian	Dale	Danby	Darcell
Cristy	Currito	Dacio	Daley	Dancer	Darcio
Crockett	Curro	Dack	Dalfon	Dandre	Darcy
Crofton	Curry	Dadrian	Dalit	Dane	Dard
Croix	Curt	Daedalus	Dallan	Daned	Dardanos
Crompton	Curtice	Daeg	Dallas	Daneil	Dardanus
Cromwell	Curtis	Daegan	Dalldav	Danek	Dare
Cronan	Curtiss	Dael	Dallen	Danel	Dareau
Cronus	Cus	Daelan	Dallin	Danelea	Dareh
Crook	Cusick	Daemon	Dallon	Danell	Darell
Crosby	Custenhin	Daemyn	Dalmazio	Dangelo	Daren
Crosley	Custodio	Dafydd	Dalon	Danger	Darence
Cross	Cuthbert	Dag	Dalton	Danhy	Darfin
Crow	Cutler	Dagan	Dalvin	Dani	Dargan
Crowell	Cutter	Dagen	Daly	Daniel	Darian
Crowther	Cuyler	Dagger	Dalyn	Daniele	Daric

Darick	Dasan	Dayne	Delaine	Demitri	Dermod
Dariel	Dash	Dayshaun	Delaire	Demitrius	Dermot
Dariell	Dashawn	Dayson	Delancy	Democracy	Dermott
Darien	Dashiell	Dayton	Delane	Demodocus	Deron
Darin	Dason	Daytona	Delaney	Demogorgon	Deronn
Dario	Dastan	Deaborn	Delano	Demonte	Derrall
Darion	Dathan	Deacon	Delany	Demophon	Derreck
Darius	Datu	Deaglan	Delaware	Demoritus	Derrek
Darko	Daube	Dean	Delbert	Demos	Derrell
Darl	Daughtry	Deance	Delbin	Demothi	Derrick
Darnel	Daulton	Deandre	Deldrach	Dempsey	Derrik
Darnell	Daumier	Deangelo	Delgado	Dempster	Derrill
Darnley	Daunte	Dearborn	Delias	Demyan	Derring
Darold	Dave	Dearg	Delius	Den	Derron
Daron	Daveigh	Deavon	Dell	Denali	Derry
Daronn	Daveney	Debonair	Delling	Denby	Derryl
Darra	Davenport	Decatur	Delmar	Denes	Derwent
Darragh	Davet	Deccan	Delmer	Denham	Derwin
Darrah	Davey	December	Delmon	Denholm	Derwyn
Darrel	Davi	Decimus	Delmont	Denim	Des
Darrell	Davian	Decker	Delmore	Denis	Descartes
Darren	David	Declan	Delmuth	Deniz	Deseronto
Darrence	Davide	Declare	Delphin	Denji	Deshan
Darrian	Davidson	Deddrick	Delray	Denley	Deshaun
Darrick	Davie	Dedrick	Delrick	Denman	Deshawn
Darrien	Davies	Dee	Delrico	Denmark	Desi
Darrin	Davignon	Deedrick	Delron	Dennet	Desiderio
Darrio	Davin	Deegan	Delroy	Dennis	Desii
Darrion	Davion	Deems	Delsaran	Dennison	Desirus
Darrius	Davionn	Deen	Delsin	Denny	Desmond
Darroch	Daviot	Deepak	Delton	Denton	Desta
Darroll	Davis	Deerick	Delvin	Denver	Destan
Darrow	Davon	Deeshawn	Delvon	Denys	Destin
Darry	Davu	Deevon	Delwin	Denzel	Destino
Darryl	Davvid	Deforest	Delwyn	Denzell	Deston
Darryll	Davyn	Dehateh	Demarco	Deo	Destrey
Darshan	Dawayne	Dei	Demarcus	Deodar	Destrie
Dart	Dawson	Deion	Demario	Deodat	Destry
Dartagnan	Dawud	Deiondre	DeMario	Deon	Detleff
Darth	Dax	Deiphobus	Demarion	Deonte	Detroit
Darthoridan	Daxon	Deiter	Demarrio	Deoradhain	Deucalion
Darton	Daxter	Dejan	Demas	Derby	Deuce
Daruka	Daxton	Dejuan	Dembe	Dereck	Deunoro
Darvell	Day	Deka	Demetre	Derek	Deus
Darvin	Dayanand	Deke	Demetri	Derell	Dev
Darwin	Daylan	Dekedrian	Demetrios	Derenik	Deva
Dary	Daylin	Dekel	Demetrius	Derex	Deval
Daryl	Daylon	Deker	Demi	Derick	Devan
Daryll	Daymon	Dekle	Demien	Derion	Devanand
Daryn	Daymond	Del	Demir	Derland	Devante

Devaughn	Dhruvesh	Dinsmore	Dome	Dontae	Drakon
Devaun	Dia	Diogenes	Domenic	Dontavius	Drannor
Deven	Diallo	Diogo	Domenico	Donte	Draper
Deveon	Diamond	Diokles	Domhnull	Dontell	Draupnir
Deveral	Dian	Diomedes	Domingo	Dontrell	Draven
Deveraux	Diandre	Dion	Dominic	Donzel	Dre
Devere	Diara	Diondre	Dominicc	Dooley	Dream
Devereau	Diarmad	Dionicio	Dominick	Doozer	Dred
Devereaux	Diarmaid	Dionizy	Dominik	Dor	Drem
Deverel	Diarmid	Dionn	Dominique	Doran	Dremidydd
Deverell	Diata	Dionte	Domino	Dorek	Drennon
Devereux	Diaz	Dionysios	Dominy	Doren	Dresden
Deverick	Dice	Dionysius	Domminic	Dorian	Drew
Deverril	Dichali	Dionysus	Domminick	Dorien	Drewes
Devery	Dick	Dior	Domo	Dorion	Drexel
Devesh	Dickinson	Diplomacy	Don	Doron	Driscol
Devin	Dickson	Dirck	Donagh	Doroteo	Driscoll
Devine	Didier	Dirk	Donahue	Dorran	Driver
Devion	Didrik	Dirrnyg	Donal	Dorrance	Drogo
Devland	Diederick	Discovery	Donald	Dorrel	Dror
Devlin	Diedrick	Divakar	Donar	Dorrell	Drover
Devlon	Diego	Diversity	Donat	Dorren	Dru
Devlyn	Diem	Divyesh	Donatello	Dorrin	Druce
Devo	Diesel	Dix	Donatien	Dorset	Drudwas
Devon	Dieter	Dixon	Donato	Dorsey	Drue
Devonte	Dietrich	Diya	Donavan	Dotson	Druindar
Devraj	Dieudonn	Django	Donaver	Doug	Drum
Devry	Digby	Djimon	Donavon	Dougal	Druman
Devven	Diggory	Dmitri	Dondre	Doughall	Drummand
Devvin	Digon	Dmitriy	Donel	Doughlas	Drummer
Devyn	Diji	Doane	Donell	Douglas	Drummond
Deward	Dilan	Dob	Dong	Douglass	Drury
Dewayne	Dillan	Dobbin	Doniel	Dougray	Druson
Dewei	Dillen	Dobbs	Donier	Dour	Drych
Dewey	Dillian	Dobieslaw	Donn	Dov	Dryden
Dewi	Dillie	Dobry	Donnacha	Dove	Drystan
Dewitt	Dillon	Doctor	Donnachadh	Dover	Dryw
Dex	Dillus	Dodek	Donnald	Dovev	Drywsone
Dexter	Dilwyn	Dodge	Donnan	Dow	Duach
Dexton	Dima	Dodson	Donnchadh	Doyle	Duald
Deylin	Dimas	Dohasan	Donne	Dracen	Duane
Dez	Dimitri	Doherty	Donnel	Drachen	Duante
Dezi	Dimka	Dohosan	Donnell	Draco	Duard
Dezso	Dimochka	Doire	Donnelly	Dracon	Duardo
Dhani	Dinand	Dolan	Donnie	Draegan	Duarte
Dharma	Dinesh	Dolph	Donnovan	Dragan	Duayne
Dhaval	Dingo	Dolphus	Donny	Drago	Dubem
Dhiren	Dinh	Dolyttle	Donough	Dragon	Dubh
Dhoire	Dino	Dom	Donovan	Drake	Dubhgan
Dhruv	Dinos	Domani	Donovann	Drakkar	Dubhglas

Dublin	Duron	Eachthighearn	Eddy	Efraim	Eirwyn
Dubois	Durothil	Eadward	Ede	Efrain	Eisa
Duc	Durrant	Eagan	Edel	Efran	Eisig
Duccio	Durrell	Eagle	Eden	Efrat	Eitan
Dudd	Durward	Eagon	Eder	Efrayim	Eja
Dude	Durwin	Ealdun	Edern	Efrem	Eka
Dudley	Durwood	Eames	Edgar	Efren	Ekewaka
Duel	Duryea	Eamon	Edgard	Efron	Eko
Duer	Dusan	Eamonn	Edgardo	Efterpi	Ekon
Duff	Duscha	Ean	Edge	Egan	Ekram
Dugald	Dushan	Eann	Edgerton	Egbert	Ekundayo
Dugan	Dusk	Eanruig	Edi	Egerton	Elad
Dughall	Dustin	Ear	Edik	Egidio	Eladio
Duha	Dusty	Earc	Edison	Egidius	Elaith
Duka	Dutch	Earie	Edisson	Egil	Elam
Duke	Duval	Earl	Edmar	Eginhard	Elan
Dulal	Duvall	Earland	Edmon	Egiodeo	Eland
Dulé	Duwayne	Earlham	Edmond	Egmont	Elandorr
Dumas	Duy	Earlston	Edmondo	Egon	Elashor
Dumi	Dvir	Early	Edmund	Egor	Elazar
Dumont	Dwade	Earnan	Edmundo	Egypt	Elazaro
Dunbar	Dwain	Earnest	Edmyg	Ehan	Elazer
Duncan	Dwaine	Earvin	Edoardo	Ehlark	Elbanco
Dundee	Dwane	Earwin	Edom	Ehren	Elbauthin
Dune	Dwayne	Earwine	Edouard	Ehrendil	Elbert
Dung	Dweezil	Earwyn	Edred	Ehud	Elbridge
Dunham	Dwi	Eastman	Edrian	Eibhear	Elchanan
Dunixi	Dwight	Easton	Edric	Eiddoel	Eldaernth
Dunley	Dwyer	Eastwood	Edsel	Eifion	Eldar
Dunlop	Dwyn	Eaton	Edson	Eike	Elden
Dunmor	Dyami	Eban	Eduard	Eilad	Elder
Dunmore	Dyer	Ebbe	Eduardo	Eiladar	Eldon
Dunn	Dyffros	Eben	Eduarte	Eilam	Eldorado
Dunne	Dyke	Ebenezer	Edvard	Eilauver	Eldred
Dunstan	Dylan	Eber	Edwald	Eilert	Eldridge
Dunton	Dyllan	Eberhard	Edwaldo	Eilian	Eldrin
Dur	Dyllon	Eberhardt	Edward	Eilif	Eldritch
Durable	Dylon	Eberlein	Edwardd	Eilig	Eldwin
Duran	Dymas	Ebisu	Edwardo	Ellis	Eleazar
Durand	Dyre	Ebner	Edwin	Eilon	Eleazer
Durango	Dyson	Ebo	Edwinn	Eilwyn	Eleftherios
Durant	Dyvynarth	Echo	Edwyrd	Eimar	Elek
Durante	Dyvyr	Eckhard	Edyrm	Eimhin	Elénaril
Durbin	Dywel	Ed	Eelia	Einar	Eleodoro
Dureau	Dzigbode	Edan	Eero	Einian	Elephon
Durell		Edbert	Eetu	Einion	Eleuterio
Durham	**E**	Eddard	Effren	Eion	Eleutherios
Durie		Eddie	Efigenio	Eire	Eleutherius
Durin	Eachan	Eddison	Efim	Eirian	Eleven
Durlan	Eachann	Eddward	Efisio	Eirik	Elford

25

Elfred	Eliya	Elul	Enan	Erasmus	Eros
Elgar	Eliyahu	Eluwilussit	Enapay	Erastus	Errapel
Elger	Eljah	Elvin	Enar	Erbin	Erric
Elgin	Elkan	Elvio	Enceladus	Ercole	Errick
Elhanan	Elkana	Elvis	Enda	Ercwlff	Errigal
Eli	Elkanah	Elvy	Ender	Erebus	Errik
Elia	Elkhazel	Elwell	Endicott	Erechtheus	Errol
Eliab	Ellair	Elwin	Endre	Erek	Erroll
Eliachim	Ellard	Elwood	Endymion	Eren	Erryn
Eliah	Ellen	Elwyn	Enea	Erendriel	Erskine
Eliakim	Ellery	Ely	Eneas	Erez	Eru
Eliam	Ellesmere	Elya	Eneco	Erglareo	Erubiel
Elian	Ellian	Elyashiv	Engel	Ergyryad	Erv
Eliana	Ellias	Emanuel	Engelbert	Erhard	Ervin
Elias	Ellijah	Emanuele	Enigma	Eri	Ervine
Eliav	Ellington	Ember	Eniola	Eric	Erving
Eliaz	Elliot	Embry	Enkoodabaoo	Ericc	Erwin
Eliazar	Elliott	Emeril	Ennio	Erichthonius	Erwyn
Elidyr	Ellis	Emerson	Ennis	Erick	Eryi
Elie	Ellisar	Emery	Eno	Erickson	Eryk
Elieis	Ellison	Emest	Enoch	Ericson	Erymanthus
Eliezer	Ellsworth	Emesto	Enos	Eridian	Erysichthon
Elif	Ellwood	Emhyr	Enrico	Erie	Eryx
Eligio	Elm	Emicho	Enrique	Erik	Esadowa
Eligius	Elman	Emil	Enriqueta	Erikk	Esai
Elihu	Elmar	Emile	Enrrique	Erikson	Esarosa
Elii	Elmer	Emilian	Ensign	Eriladar	Esau
Eliijah	Elmo	Emiliano	Ensio	Erin	Esav
Elija	Elmore	Emilien	Entrydal	Eriq	Esben
Elijaah	Elnadav	Emilio	Enyeto	Erix	Esbjorn
Elijah	Elnatan	Emilliano	Enzo	Eriyn	Eschallus
Elijahh	Elod	Emillio	Enzzo	Erlan	Escott
Elijha	Elof	Emir	Eoghan	Erland	Esdras
Elimelech	Eloi	Emlyn	Eoin	Erlathan	Esequiel
Elio	Elois	Emlen	Eónan	Erlend	Eshkol
Elioenai	Elon	Emlyn	Epaminondas	Erling	Esias
Elion	Elorshin	Emmanuel	Epeius	Ermanno	Eskander
Elior	Eloy	Emmanuele	Epemetheus	Ermen	Eske
Eliot	Elpaerae	Emmet	Ephah	Ermenegildo	Eskel
Eliott	Elphin	Emmett	Ephai	Ermid	Eskil
Eliphalet	Elpidos	Emmilian	Ephraim	Ermin	Esmail
Eliron	Elrad	Emmiliano	Ephram	Ernan	Esme
Elisee	Elroy	Emmitt	Ephrath	Ernest	Esmond
Eliseo	Elsdon	Emmons	Ephrem	Ernesto	Espen
Elisha	Elson	Emmyth	Ephron	Ernie	Espn
Elishama	Elstan	Emo	Epicurus	Erno	Esra
Elisheba	Elston	Emory	Epifanio	Ernst	Essery
Elisheva	Elsu	Emrys	Eracio	Eroan	Essex
Elisud	Eltaor	Emsley	Eran	Erolith	Essien
Eliud	Elton	Emyr	Erasmo	Eron	Estanislao

Este	Euroa	Evyatar	Faddei	Falkner	Farzad	
Esteban	Euros	Evyn	Fadey	Fallon	Fate	
Estefan	Eurus	Evzen	Fadeyka	Fallows	Fateh	
Estelar	Euryalus	Ewald	Fadeyushka	Falmouth	Fathi	
Estes	Eurylochus	Ewan	Fadi	Fane	Fathih	
Estevan	Eurymachus	Ewart	Fadil	Fanuco	Faulkner	
Estevao	Eurypylus	Ewen	Fadile	Faodhagan	Faunus	
Estevon	Eurystheus	Ewert	Fadri	Faolan	Faust	
Estienne	Euryton	Ewing	Fadyenka	Farah	Fausto	
Eston	Eus	Exodus	Faegan	Faraj	Faustus	
Etan	Eusebius	Experience	Faelar	Faraji	Favian	
Etchemin	Eustace	Explorer	Faelyn	Faramond	Favorite	
Eteocles	Eustachy	Eyad	Faer	Faraz	Favre	
Ethan	Eustatius	Eyal	Faeranduil	Fardoragh	Fawzi	
Ethanael	Eustis	Eyoel	Faerwald	Fares	Faxon	
Ethaniel	Euston	Eyolf	Fafner	Fargo	Fay	
Ethann	Evaan	Eyou	Fagan	Farhad	Fayette	
Ethelbert	Evan	Eyrynnhv	Fagen	Farid	Fayiz	
Ethelred	Evander	Eytan	Fagin	Faris	Feandan	
Ethelwin	Evangel	Ezechiel	Fahd	Farlan	Fearchar	
Ethelwulf	Evann	Ezekial	Fahey	Farlane	Fearghus	
Ethen	Evans	Ezekiel	Fahim	Farley	February	
Ethlando	Evarado	Ezell	Fahroni	Farmer	Fechin	
Etienne	Evardo	Ezequiel	Fahy	Farnell	Fedde	
Etlelooaat	Evaristus	Ezer	Fai	Farnham	Fedele	
Etor	Evea	Ezhno	Fallon	Farnley	Federico	
Ettore	Evelyn	Ezio	Fain	Faro	Fedor	
Ettrian	Even	Ezra	Faine	Farold	Fedya	
Etu	Ever	Ezrah	Faing	Faron	Fedyenka	
Etzel	Everard	Eztli	Fairbairn	Farouk	Feeny	
Euan	Everardo		Fairbanks	Farquahar	Feivel	
Eubuleus	Everest	**F**	Fairchild	Farquhar	Felaern	
Euclid	Everett		Fairfax	Farquharson	Felan	
Eudav	Everhart	Faas	Fairly	Farr	Feleti	
Eudocio	Everild	Fabi	Faisal	Farrah	Felician	
Eugen	Everley	Fabian	Faivish	Farran	Feliciano	
Eugene	Everly	Fabiano	Faiz	Farrar	Felicien	
Eugenio	Evers	Fabien	Fajr	Farrel	Felicio	
Eugenios	Evert	Fabio	Fakhir	Farrell	Feliks	
Eugenius	Everton	Fabion	Fakhiri	Farren	Felim	
Eulogio	Evgeni	Fabius	Fakhri	Farrin	Felinus	
Eumaeus	Evgenii	Fable	Falael	Farris	Felipe	
Eunan	Evgeniy	Fabrice	Falan	Farrokh	Felippe	
Euodias	Evian	Fabrico	Falco	Farrow	Felix	
Eupeithes	Evin	Fabrizio	Falcon	Farrs	Fell	
Euphemios	Evindal	Fabron	Falconer	Farruco	Fellipe	
Euphrates	Evo	Fabumi	Faldo	Fars	Felton	
Euphrosyne	Evon	Fachnan	Falito	Farson	Fenian	
Eurion	Evoy	Fachtna	Falk	Faruq	Fenmore	
Euripides	Evrawg	Factor	Falke	Farvardin	Fenn	

Fennel	Fiero	Fitzgerald	Foma	Frandscus	Friday
Fenno	Fife	Fitzhugh	Fonda	Frandszk	Fridolf
Fenris	Fifer	Fitzroy	Fone	Frang	Fridolph
Fenton	Figueroa	Fitzwilliam	Fonso	Frank	Friduwulf
Feo	Filarion	Flynn	Fontaine	Frankie	Fridwolf
Feodor	Filbert	Fjodor	Fontana	Frankito	Friedrich
Feodras	Filiberto	Flaco	Fontane	Franklin	Friend
Feoras	Filip	Flainn	Fontayne	Franklyn	Frigyes
Fercos	Filippo	Flame	Fonteyne	Franky	Frisco
Ferdinand	Filips	Flan	Fonzell	Frannsaidh	Friso
Ferdinando	Fillip	Flanagan	Fonzie	Frans	Frits
Ferenc	Filmore	Flanders	Fonzo	Franz	Fritz
Fergal	Filvendor	Flann	Forba	Franziskus	Fritzi
Fergall	Filverel	Flannagain	Forbes	Frasco	Frode
Fergie	Finbar	Flannerry	Ford	Frascuelo	Frodi
Fergus	Finch	Flannery	Fordon	Fraser	Frodo
Ferguson	Findlay	Flardryn	Foreman	Frasier	Frost
Feri	Fineen	Flash	Forest	Frayne	Fryderyk
Ferke	Finesse	Flavian	Forester	Frazer	Frye
Ferlin	Fingal	Flavio	Forestt	Frazier	Fuentes
Fermin	Finian	Flavius	Forever	Fred	Fuji
Fernand	Finlay	Flawiusz	Forrest	Fredderick	Fulbright
Fernando	Finley	Fleet	Forrester	Freddie	Fulk
Ferrari	Finn	Fleetwood	Forrestt	Freddrick	Fuller
Ferrell	Finnbar	Fleming	Forseti	Freddy	Fulop
Ferris	Finnegan	Fletcher	Forster	Fredek	Fulton
Ferrol	Finnian	Flin	Fort	Frederek	Fursey
Festus	Finnick	Flinar	Fortino	Frederic	Future
Fews	Finnigan	Flinn	Fortitude	Frederick	Fychan
Fferyll	Finnin	Flint	Fortney	Frederico	Fylson
Fflergant	Finnlay	Flip	Fortun	Fredrick	Fynbar
Fflewdwr	Finnobarr	Floi	Fortune	Fredrik	Fynn
Ffodor	Fionan	Floinn	Fortuo	Free	Fyodor
Ffowc	Fionn	Florent	Forum	Freeborn	Fyrsil
Fhaornik	Fionnbarr	Florentijn	Foster	Freed	
Fiachra	Fionnlagh	Florentino	Fountain	Freedom	
Fiacre	Fiorello	Florian	Fowler	Freeman	**G**
Flannan	Fiorenzo	Florin	Fox	Freman	
Fibh	Fire	Florinio	Foxfire	Fremont	
Fico	Firman	Florus	Foy	French	Gaagii
Fidal	Firth	Floyd	Fraco	Frenchie	Gaane
Fidel	Firuz	Flurin	Fraley	Frenchy	Gabai
Fidele	Fischer	Flurry	Fran	Freowine	Gabato
Fidelio	Fishel	Flyn	Francesco	Fresco	Gabbo
Fidelis	Fisher	Flynn	Franchot	Frewin	Gabe
Fidello	Fisk	Flynt	Francis	Frewyn	Gabek
Fie	Fiske	Fnam	Francisco	Frey	Gabi
Field	Fisseha	Fogarty	Franco	Freyr	Gabian
Fielder	Fitch	Foley	Francois	Frici	Gabie
Fielding	Fitz	Folke	François	Frick	Gabin

Gabino	Galeno	Gardener	Garve	Gearoid	Geovanni
Gable	Galeun	Gardiner	Garvey	Geary	Geovanny
Gabo	Gali	Gardner	Garvin	Gedalia	Geovany
Gabor	Galil	Gare	Garwood	Gedaliah	Geraint
Gabrian	Galilee	Gared	Garwyli	Gedalya	Gerald
Gabriel	Galileo	Garen	Gary	Gedalyahu	Geraldo
Gabriele	Galinthias	Garet	Garynnon	Geddes	Geralt
Gabrielo	Gall	Gareth	Gascon	Gedeon	Gerard
Gabrio	Gallagher	Garett	Gaspar	Geert	Gerardo
Gabryle	Gallatin	Garfield	Gaspard	Geet	Gerasim
Gace	Gallio	Garian	Gaston	Gefen	Gerben
Gad	Galloway	Garin	Gates	Geffrey	Gerek
Gadhi	Galo	Garion	Gatik	Gehrig	Geremia
Gadhra	Galt	Garlan	Gatland	Gehry	Gergely
Gadi	Galtem	Garland	Gatlin	Geir	Gergo
Gadiel	Galterio	Garlen	Gatsby	Gelasius	Gergor
Gadish	Galtero	Garlyn	Gattaca	Gellert	Gerhard
Gael	Galton	Garman	Gaubert	Gemi	Gerik
Gaelan	Galvin	Garnell	Gauge	Gemini	Gerlach
Gaeleath	Galvyn	Garner	Gauguin	Genaro	Germain
Gaelin	Galway	Garnet	Gaurav	Gene	Germaine
Gaerwn	Galyn	Garnett	Gautam	Genero	German
Gaery	Gamada	Garnoc	Gauthier	Generosb	Germano
Gaetan	Gamal	Garnock	Gautier	Genesis	Germanus
Gaetano	Gamaliel	Garon	Gav	Genet	Gerodi
Gagan	Gamble	Garrad	Gavan	Genius	Gerome
Gage	Gamliel	Garran	Gaven	Genkei	Geron
Gahan	Ganamede	Garrard	Gavi	Gennadi	Geronimo
Gahiji	Gandhi	Garren	Gavin	Gennadiy	Gerontius
Gaige	Gandolf	Garret	Gavinn	Gennaro	Gerrald
Gaile	Gandy	Garreth	Gavino	Gent	Gerrard
Gaillard	Ganesa	Garrett	Gavivi	Gentian	Gerred
Gainell	Ganesh	Garrey	Gavrel	Gentile	Gerrell
Gaines	Ganger	Garrick	Gavrie	Gentry	Gerrit
Gair	Ganit	Garridan	Gavriel	Genty	Gerritt
Gairbhith	Gannet	Garrik	Gavriil	Geoff	Gerrod
Gairbith	Gannon	Garrin	Gavril	Geoffrey	Gerry
Gaius	Gantar	Garrison	Gavrilovich	Geoffroi	Gersham
Gajijens	Ganya	Garritt	Gavvin	Geomar	Gershom
Gal	Ganymede	Garron	Gawain	Gcona	Gershon
Galaeron	Gar	Garroway	Gavynn	Geordi	Gershwin
Galahad	Gara	Garrson	Gawain	Georg	Gerson
Galal	Garan	Garry	Gawen	George	Gervais
Galan	Garanhon	Garson	Gawyn	Georges	Gervaise
Galather	Garanwyn	Garsone	Gay	Georgi	Gervase
Galaxy	Garbhach	Garsteaode	Gaylen	Georgie	Gervasio
Galbraith	Garbhan	Garth	Gaylord	Georgino	Gervaso
Galchobhar	Garcia	Garton	Gaynor	Georgio	Gerwazy
Gale	Gard	Garuda	Gazali	Georgiy	Gery
Galen	Gardar	Garvan	Gearald	Geovani	Gethin

Gethsemane	Gillett	Gladwin	Gomer	Gowyr	Gregori
Gevariah	Gilli	Glaleanna	Gonen	Graceland	Gregoria
Gezane	Gillies	Glanville	Gonzalo	Gracia	Gregorie
Ghaith	Gillis	Glarald	Goodman	Graciana	Gregorio
Ghaleb	Gilman	Glasgow	Goodwin	Graciano	Gregorior
Ghalib	Gilmer	Glaucio	Goodwine	Graddy	Gregory
Ghassan	Gilmore	Glaucus	Goodwyn	Gradin	Gregos
Ghayth	Gilon	Gleb	Goodyear	Gradon	Greid
Ghazi	Gilroy	Gleen	Gopi	Grady	Grendel
Ghoukas	Gilson	Gleipnif	Gopinath	Graeae	Grenier
Giacomo	Gilvaethwy	Gleis	Goraidh	Graeme	Grenville
Gian	Gimle	Glen	Goran	Graham	Gresham
Giancarlo	Ginebra	Glenavon	Gorane	Grahame	Greville
Gianncarlo	Ginessa	Glendon	Gordain	Grail	Grey
Giannes	Ginjiro	Glendower	Gordan	Gram	Greydon
Gianni	Ginno	Glenn	Gordie	Gramercy	Greyson
Gib	Gino	Glenville	Gordon	Granger	Grian
Gibbes	Giolla	Glenward	Gordy	Granite	Gridley
Gibor	Giomar	Glew	Gore	Grant	Griff
Gibson	Giona	Glinyeu	Goren	Grantham	Griffen
Giddeon	Giorgio	Glorandal	Goreu	Grantland	Griffeth
Gide	Giotto	Glover	Gorham	Grantley	Griffey
Gideon	Giovani	Glyn	Gorka	Granville	Griffin
Gidja	Giovanii	Glynn	Gorky	Granwen	Griffith
Gidon	Giovanni	Gnash	Gorman	Grathgor	Grigor
Giffard	Giovanny	Gnegon	Gormant	Gratian	Grigori
Gifford	Giovany	Gobind	Goro	Graves	Grigorii
Gift	Giovonni	Gobrwy	Gorou	Gray	Grigoriy
Gig	Gipsy	Godalupe	Gorrell	Graydan	Grigorov
Gijs	Girisha	Godana	Gorrie	Grayden	Grigory
Gijsbert	Girolamo	Goddard	Gorry	Graydon	Grim
Gil	Girven	Godewyn	Gorsedd	Grayer	Grimaldo
Gilad	Girvin	Godfredo	Gorton	Graysen	Grimshaw
Gilam	Girvyn	Godfrey	Gosheven	Grayson	Grimsley
Gilbert	Gisli	Godfried	Gotham	Grayton	Grioghar
Gilberto	Gitana	Godofredo	Gothfraidh	Graziano	Griorgair
Gilby	Gitano	Godric	Gottfrid	Greagoir	Grisha
Gilchrist	Giuliano	Godwin	Gottfried	Greco	Griswold
Gilead	Giulio	Godwine	Gotthard	Greeley	Grosvenor
Giles	Giullio	Godwyn	Gotzone	Green	Grove
Gilfred	Giuseppe	Gofraidh	Gough	Greenlee	Grover
Gili	Giustino	Gofried	Gov	Greenwood	Gru
Gill	Glyn	Gogol	Govan	Greer	Gruddyeu
Gillanders	Glynn	Gokmen	Govannon	Greg	Gruev
Gille	Gizeh	Goku	Govert	Greger	Gruffen
Gillean	Gizur	Golden	Govind	Gregg	Gruffin
Gilleasbuig	Gjorn	Golding	Gow	Greggory	Gruffudd
Gillermo	Glacier	Goldsmith	Gowan	Gregoire	Gruffyn
Gilles	Glade	Goldwin	Gower	Gregoly	Grufydd
Gillespie	Gladstone	Goliath	Gowyn	Gregor	Gryphin

Gryphon	Guto	Habakkuk	Halafarin	Hamisi	Hardy
Guadalupe	Guttorm	Haben	Halamar	Hamlet	Harel
Guadelupe	Guy	Habib	Halbert	Hamlin	Harford
Gualterio	Guyapi	Habiki	Halcyon	Hammad	Hargrove
Gualtier	Guylan	Hachi	Haldan	Hammer	Hari
Gualtiero	Guzman	Hachiro	Halden	Hammet	Haris
Guang	Gwakhmai	Hachirou	Haldis	Hammett	Harischandra
Guban	Gwalchmai	Hackett	Haldor	Hammond	Harith
Guerrant	Gwalchmei	Hackman	Haldreithen	Hampden	Harkahome
Guglielmo	Gwalhaved	Haco	Hale	Hampton	Harkin
Gui	Gwallawg	Hadar	Halen	Hampus	Harlan
Guido	Gwallter	Haddad	Haley	Hamund	Harlem
Guifford	Gwarthegydd	Hadden	Halflar	Hamza	Harlequin
Guildford	Gwawl	Haden	Halford	Hamzah	Harley
Guilio	Gwayne	Hades	Hali	Hanan	Harlon
Guillaume	Gweir	Hadi	Halia	Hancock	Harlow
Guillelmina	Gwenael	Hadley	Halian	Handel	Harm
Guillem	Gwern	Hadrian	Halifax	Hanes	Harman
Guillermo	Gwernach	Hadriel	Halil	Hanford	Harme
Guitain	Gwevyl	Hadrien	Halim	Hani	Harmen
Guitar	Gwilenhin	Hadwin	Halirrhothius	Hania	Harmon
Gul	Gwilym	Hael	Halithersis	Hanif	Harmony
Gull	Gwitart	Haemir	Hall	Hanish	Harold
Gulliver	Gwrddywal	Haemon	Hallam	Hank	Haroun
Gulshan	Gwres	Hafez	Hallan	Hanley	Harp
Gulzar	Gwyddawg	Hafgrim	Hallberg	Hannah	Harper
Gunesh	Gwydion	Hafiz	Halle	Hannes	Harpo
Gunn	Gwydre	Hagan	Halley	Hannibal	Harpocrates
Gunnar	Gwydyon	Hagar	Halliwell	Hanno	Harrell
Gunner	Gwylym	Hagen	Hallmar	Hanns	Harrington
Gunnolf	Gwyn	Hagibis	Halloran	Hanoch	Harris
Gunny	Gwynedd	Hagley	Hallward	Hans	Harrison
Gunter	Gwyngad	Hagop	Halsey	Hansel	Harrod
Günter	Gwynn	Hagrid	Halstead	Hansen	Harrold
Gunther	Gwyr	Hahnee	Halston	Hanson	Harry
Gur	Gwystyl	Haidar	Halton	Hansraj	Harshad
Guri	Gwythyr	Haiden	Halueth	Hanzila	Hart
Gurion	Gyala	Haig	Halueve	Hao	Harta
Gurnam	Gyan	Hailama	Halvard	Happy	Harte
Guryon	Gyes	Haim	Halvor	Harailt	Hartford
Gus	Gyoergy	Haines	Halyn	Harald	Hartigan
Gusg	Gyorgy	Hajari	Ham	Harb	Hartley
Gustaof	Gyula	Haji	Hamal	Harbin	Hartley
Gustav	Gyuri	Hakan	Hamar	Harbor	Hartman
Gustava		Hakeem	Hamed	Harcourt	Hartmann
Gustave	**H**	Hakim	Hamid	Harden	Hartmut
Gustavo		Hakizimana	Hamidi	Harding	Harto
Gustavus	Haaken	Hakon	Hamill	Hardouin	Hartwell
Gusty	Haakon	Hal	Hamilton	Hardwick	Hartwig
Guthrie	Haavard	Haladavar	Hamish	Hardwin	Haru

31

Harue	Hayley	Henderson	Hershel	Hinata	Homar
Haruki	Haytham	Hendrick	Hertz	Hinto	Homare
Harun	Hayward	Hendrik	Hertzel	Hippolyte	Homayoun
Haruni	Haywood	Hendrix	Herve	Hippolytus	Homer
Haruto	Hayyim	Henley	Herzl	Hiraku	Homeros
Harvard	Hazael	Henning	Hesed	Hiral	Homerus
Harvey	Hazaiah	Hennry	Heskovizenako	Hiram	Hommer
Harvir	Hazard	Henoch	Hesperos	Hiro	Homobono
Harwood	Haze	Henri	Hesutu	Hiroaki	Honani
Haryk	Hazelton	Henrich	Hevataneo	Hiroshi	Honaw
Hasad	Hazen	Henrick	Hevel	Hiroto	Honesto
Hasani	Hazleton	Henrik	Hewett	Hiroyoshi	Hongvi
Hashem	Hazlewood	Henriqua	Hewitt	Hiroyuki	Honi
Hashim	Heammawihio	Henrique	Hewney	Hirsi	Honon
Hasim	Heardind	Henrry	Hewson	History	Honor
Hasin	Heath	Henry	Heywood	Hitch	Honoratas
Haskal	Heathcliff	Henryk	Hezekiah	Hitchcock	Honorato
Haskall	Heaton	HenWas	Hiamovi	Hiyan	Honore
Haskel	Heber	HenWyneb	Hiawatha	Hizkiyahu	Honoria
Haskell	Hector	Hephaestus	Hibine	Hjalmar	Honovi
Haslett	Hedd	Heracles	Hid	Hoai	Hooker
Hassan	Heddwyn	Heraclio	Hidalgo	Hoang	Hooper
Hassel	Hedeon	Heraklesr	Hideaki	Hob	Hoover
Hassun	Hedley	Herald	Hideki	Hobart	Hoowanneka
Hastiin	Hedwig	Herb	Hideo	Hobbes	Hopeton
Hastin	Hehu	Herbert	Hideyoshi	Hobson	Hopkins
Hastings	Heike	Herbst	Hien	Hoccar	Hopper
Hastos	Heilyn	Hercule	Hieremias	Hockley	Horace
Hatharal	Heimdall	Hercules	Hiero	Hockney	Horado
Havana	Heimrich	Heremon	Hieronim	Hod	Horatio
Håvard	Heinrich	Hereward	Hieronymos	Hodgson	Horemheb
Havelock	Heinroch	Heribert	Hieronymous	Hodor	Horith
Haven	Heinz	Heriberto	Hieronymus	Hoffman	Horizon
Havika	Hekli	Herman	Hieu	Hogan	Horrace
Hawaii	Heladio	Hermann	Hikaru	Hokaratcha	Horsley
Haward	Helaku	Hermes	Hikmat	Hoku	Horst
Hawes	Helge	Hermod	Hilaire	Holbrook	Hortencia
Hawiovi	Helgi	Hermosa	Hilal	Holcomb	Horton
Hawk	Helio	Hernan	Hilario	Holdan	Horus
Hawkins	Helios	Hernandez	Hilary	Holden	Hosa
Hawley	Helki	Hernando	Hildebrand	Holdon	Hosea
Hawthorne	Helladius	Herndon	Hildefuns	Holiday	Hosei
Hay	Heller	Herne	Hill	Hollace	Hoshea
Hayate	Helmfried	Hernley	Hillard	Holland	Hotah
Hayato	Helmut	Hero	Hillary	Holleb	Hotaka
Hayden	Helsinki	Herodotus	Hillel	Hollis	Hotaru
Haydn	Helushka	Herold	Hilliard	Holly	Hototo
Haydon	Heman	Heron	Hilol	Holman	Houghton
Haye	HEMI	Herrick	Hilton	Holmes	Houman
Hayes	Hemingway	Herschel	Himesh	Holt	Houston

Hovan	Humvee	Iaokim	Ignacio	Ilya	Innocenzio
Hovannes	Hung	Iapetus	Ignado	Ilyas	Inocencio
Hoven	Hunt	Iasion	Ignat	Imad	Inocente
Hovhaness	Hunter	Iason	Ignatius	Imagine	Inoke
Hovsep	Huntington	Iau	Ignatz	Iman	Insula
Howahkan	Huntley	Ib	Ignazio	Imani	Inteus
Howard	Huntter	Iban	Igone	Imanol	Intevar
Howe	Huon	Ibis	Igor	Imaran	Inver
Howea	Huracan	Ibo	Igorr	Imari	Inys
Howel	Huritt	Ibrahim	Igoryok	Immanol	Ioakim
Howell	Hurlbert	Ibsen	Ihab	Immanuel	Ioan
Howi	Hurley	Ibycus	Ihaka	Imran	Ioanis
Howie	Hurst	Icarius	Ihu	Imre	Iokua
Howland	Husam	Icarus	Ihuicatl	Imri	Iolani
Hoyt	Husani	Ice	Ike	Imtiyaz	Iolas
Hrimfaxi	Huslu	Icelos	Ikee	Inachus	Iolo
Hrolleif	Hussein	Ichabod	Iker	Inali	Iolrath
Hrut	Huston	Ichiro	Ikerne	Inay	Ion
Hu	Hutchings	Ichirou	Ikram	Ince	Iona
Huabwy	Hutchinson	Ichtaca	Iku	Incendio	Ionakana
Huarwar	Hutton	Ickett	Ilan	Incenio	Ionnes
Hubbard	Huw	Ickitt	Ilar	Inchel	Iorgas
Hubbell	Huxford	Icnoyotl	Ilara	Increase	Iorwerth
Hubbert	Huxley	Icos	Ilari	Indiana	Iosef
Hubert	Huy	Ida	Ilario	Indigo	Iosep
Hubie	Hy	Idal	Ilbryn	Indio	Ioseph
Hubyr	Hyacinth	Idan	Ileanna	Indivar	Iov
Huck	Hyacinthe	Idas	Ilham	Indra	Ioviano
Huckleberry	Hyatt	Iddawg	Iliana	Indus	Iowereth
Hud	Hydd	Iddig	Ilias	Indy	Iphicrates
Hudd	Hyde	Iden	Ilie	Inerney	Iphitus
Hudson	Hyder	Idi	Ilima	Infinity	Ipo
Hueil	Hyman	Ido	Ilimitar	Ingemar	Iqbal
Huey	Hyperion	Idoia	Iliphar	Inglebert	Ira
Huffington	Hypnos	Idomeneus	Iliya	Ingmar	Iraia
Hugh	Hyroniemus	Idris	Ilkay	Ingo	Iraj
Hughie	Hywel	Idurre	Illan	Ingram	Iram
Hughson		Iefyr	Illanipi	Ingvar	Ireland
Hugi	**I**	Ieuan	Illianaro	Ini-herit	Irem
Hugin		Ievos	Illias	Iniabi	Irenio
Hugo	Iaan	Ifan	Illinois	Inialos	Iresh
Hugues	Iago	Ifor	Illithor	Inigo	Irfan
Hui	Iain	Igasho	Illitran	Iniko	Irish
Hula	Iakona	Igashu	Ilo	Inis	Irus
Hulbert	Iakopa	Ige	Ilom	Iniss	Irvin
Humbert	Iakovos	Iggi	Ilori	Injros	Irving
Humberto	Ian	Iggy	Ilphas	Inman	Irwin
Hume	Iann	Igme	Ilrune	Innes	Isa
Hummer	Ianto	Ignace	Ilthuryn	Innis	Isaac
Humphrey	Ianu	Ignacia	Ily	Innocent	Isaak

Isaakios	Itai	Izel	Jacobson	Jahiem	Jamarion
Isadore	Italo	Izeyah	Jacobus	Jahmar	Jamarr
Isadoro	Itamar	Izidor	Jacoby	Jahnu	Jamarri
Isah	Ithaca	Izod	Jacop	Jai	Jamaun
Isai	Itham	Izreal	Jacorey	Jaidden	Jame
Isaiah	Itiel	Izzaiah	Jacory	Jaiden	Jameel
Isaias	Itotia	Izzy	Jacot	Jaidenn	Jamel
Isaie	Itsuki		Jacquan	Jaiiden	James
Isam	Ittamar	**J**	Jacque	Jaime	Jamese
Isamu	Itzak		Jacqueleen	Jaimenacho	Jameson
Isandro	Iulio	Jaaden	Jacquelin	Jaimin	Jamess
Isdel	Iustig	Jaafan	Jacques	Jaimini	Jamesson
Iseabail	Ivaan	Jaalen	Jacquez	Jain	Jamian
Iser	Ivailo	Jaan	Jacy	Jair	Jamie
Ishaan	Ivan	Jaap	Jad	Jaira	Jamiel
Isham	Ivanhoe	Jaaron	Jada	Jairdan	Jamieson
Ishaq	Ivankor	Jaason	Jade	Jairo	Jamil
Ishedus	Ivann	Jaavon	Jaden	Jairus	Jamill
Ishmael	Ivano	Jabari	Jader	Jaison	Jamin
Isi	Ivar	Jabarl	Jadiel	Jaivin	Jamir
Isiah	Iven	Jabarri	Jadon	Jajaun	Jamison
Isidor	Iver	Jabbar	Jadrian	Jaka	Jammar
Isidore	Ives	Jabez	Jadrien	Jake	Jammel
Isidoro	Ivey	Jabilo	Jadyn	Jakeem	Jammes
Isidro	Ivlisar	Jabin	Jae	Jakeson	Jamon
Iskander	Ivo	Jabir	Jaeden	Jakkob	Jamshid
Islam	Ivor	Jabr	Jaedon	Jakob	Jamya
Isley	Ivory	Jabre	Jaegar	Jakobe	Jan
Ismael	Ivósaar	Jabril	Jaeger	Jakobee	Janah
Ismail	Ivran	Jabulani	Jael	Jakome	Janak
Ismat	Ivri	Jac	Jaetyn	Jakub	Janardan
Ismet	Ivrit	Jacan	Jafar	Jaladhi	Jancsi
Isocrates	Iwalani	Jaccob	Jafari	Jalal	Jandar
Isra	Iwan	Jace	Jafaru	Jalen	Janek
Israel	Iwatoke	Jacek	Jaffar	Jalenn	Janesh
Isreal	Iwdael	Jacey	Jaffer	Jalil	Jani
Isrrael	Ixaka	Jachai	Jag	Jallen	Janie
Issa	Ixion	Jachin	Jagannath	Jalmari	Janison
Issac	Ixtli	Jacinto	Jagat	Jam	Jankia
Issachar	Iyar	Jack	Jager	Jamaal	Janko
Issai	Iye	Jackie	Jagger	Jamaar	Janli
Issaiah	Iymbryl	Jackopa	Jagmeet	Jamaari	Janna
Issaias	Iyrandrar	Jackson	Jago	Jamael	Jannalor
Issay	Izaak	Jacky	Jaguar	Jamaica	Janne
Issey	Izaiah	Jaco	Jagur	Jamal	Jannes
Istaqa	Izak	Jacob	Jahan	Jamar	Jannick
Istu	Izar	Jacobb	Jahdahdieh	Jamarcus	Jannik
Istvan	Izayah	Jacobe	Jaheem	Jamareon	Janos
Ita	Ize	Jacobean	Jaheim	Jamari	Janson
Itachi	Izek	Jacobo	Jahi	Jamarii	Jantje

34

Jantzen	Jarren	Jayce	Jeff	Jeremie	Jerzyr
Januarius	Jarret	Jaycee	Jefferey	Jeremmy	Jesiah
January	Jarrett	Jayceon	Jefferson	Jeremy	Jesimiel
Janus	Jarrod	Jaycob	Jeffery	Jeren	Jesper
Janyd	Jarron	Jaydden	Jefford	Jerett	Jess
Janyl	Jarvis	Jaydee	Jeffrey	Jeriah	Jessamine
Jaonos	Jas	Jayden	Jeffry	Jericho	Jesse
Japhet	Jascha	Jaydon	Jehoiakim	Jerico	Jessen
Japheth	Jase	Jaye	Jehoichin	Jeriel	Jessey
Japhy	Jasen	Jayin	Jehu	Jermain	Jessie
Jaquan	Jaser	Jaylan	Jeirgif	Jermaine	Jesstin
Jaques	Jasha	Jaylen	Jela	Jermajesty	Jessus
Jaquez	Jasiah	Jaylin	Jelle	Jermey	Jessy
Jarad	Jasiel	Jayllen	Jem	Jermija	Jestin
Jarah	Jasleen	Jaylon	Jemal	Jeroboam	Jeston
Jaran	Jasmin	Jayme	Jemuel	Jerod	Jesualdo
Jardine	Jason	Jaymes	Jencir	Jeroen	Jesus
Jareb	Jasonn	Jaymin	Jenda	Jeroenr	Jet
Jared	Jaspar	Jaymz	Jengo	Jerold	Jeter
Jaredd	Jasper	Jayr	Jenkin	Jerom	Jethro
Jarek	Jassin	Jayron	Jenner	Jerome	Jetson
Jarel	Jasson	Jayse	Jennis	Jeromee	Jett
Jarell	Jathan	Jaysen	Jeno	Jeron	Jeven
Jaren	Jati	Jayson	Jens	Jeronimo	Jevin
Jaret	Jatin	Jayvee	Jensen	Jerrad	Jevon
Jareth	Java	Jayvon	Jenski	Jerrah	Jevonn
Jarett	Javan	Jayvonn	Jenson	Jerrald	Jevonte
Jari	Javana	Jayyed	Jenue	Jerrall	Jex
Jariah	Javed	Jaz	Jeny	Jerramie	Jhaan
Jariath	Javelin	Jazmina	Jeoffroi	Jerramy	Jhaartael
Jarin	Javen	Jazz	Jeor	Jerred	Jhaeros
Jarini	Javes	Jean	Jephtah	Jerrell	Jharak
Jarius	Javier	Jean Baptiste	Jephthah	Jerremiah	Jharym
Jarl	Javiero	JeanBaptiste	Jeppe	Jerremy	Jiang
Jarlan	Javion	Jeb	Jerad	Jerren	Jibri
Jarlath	Javon	Jebediah	Jerah	Jerrett	Jibril
Jarmaine	Javonn	Jed	Jerald	Jerric	Jicarilla
Jarman	Javonte	Jedadiah	Jeraldo	Jerricho	Jie
Jarod	Jawanza	Jedaiah	Jerall	Jerrick	Jihan
Jarom	Jawdat	Jedd	Jerard	Jerrin	Jiles
Jaromir	Jax	Jedediah	Jerardo	Jerrod	Jim
Jaron	Jaxen	Jedi	Jere	Jerrold	Jimbo
Jaronn	Jaxith	Jediah	Jered	Jerrome	Jimi
Jaroslav	Jaxon	Jedidiah	Jerel	Jerron	Jimm
Jarrad	Jaxson	Jedrek	Jerell	Jerry	Jimmie
Jarrah	Jaxton	Jedrick	Jereme	Jersey	Jimmy
Jarran	Jaxx	Jedrik	Jeremey	Jerusalem	Jinan
Jarred	Jaxxon	Jedrus	Jeremi	Jervis	Jinendra
Jarrel	Jaxxson	Jedrzej	Jeremiah	Jeryl	Jinjur
Jarrell	Jay	Jeevan	Jeremias	Jerzy	Jinx

Jirair	Johnson	Jordy	Jourdan	Jun	Kabos
Jiri	Jojen	Jordyn	Jourdon	Junaid	Kacey
Jirkar	Jokin	Jore	Journey	Junayd	Kachada
Jiro	Jokkum	Jorell	Jov	Juneau	Kadar
Jirou	Jokull	Joren	Jovaan	Jung	Kaddish
Jiva	Jolie	Jorenr	Jovan	Junien	Kade
Jivan	Jollie	Jorg	Jovani	Junior	Kadeem
Jivin	Jolon	Jorge	Jovanni	Juniper	Kaden
Jo	Jolyon	Jorgen	Jovany	Junipero	Kader
Joab	Jomar	Jørgen	Jove	Junius	Kadin
Joachim	Jomei	Jori	Joweese	Juno	Kadir
Joah	Jon	Jorian	Joy	Junot	Kadmiel
Joakim	Jonah	Jorie	Joyanna	Junpei	Kadmus
Joan	Jonam	Jorildyn	Joyce	Jupiter	Kaeden
Joao	Jonas	Jorim	Joyner	Juppar	Kael
Joaquin	Jonatan	Joris	Joziah	Jurg	Kaelan
Joash	Jonathan	Jormungand	Jozsef	Jurgen	Kaelem
Job	Jonathon	Jorn	Juan	Jurgisr	Kaelin
Joban	Jonattan	Jorrin	Juan-Carlos	Juri	Kaemon
Jobe	Jonatthan	Jorryn	Juancho	Juriaan	Kafele
Joben	Jonco	Jory	Juanito	Juro	Kafka
Joby	Jondalar	Jos	Juaquine	Jurou	Kaga
Jocelin	Jones	Jose	Jubal	Jurre	Kagan
Jocelyn	Jonesy	Joseba	Jud	Jurrijn	Kagiso
Jocheved	Jonik	Josef	Judaea	Jussi	Kahlil
Jock	Jonn	Joseff	Judah	Juste	Kahn
Jodee	Jonnatan	Joselito	Judas	Justice	Kahoku
Jody	Jonnathan	Josep	Judd	Justin	Kai
Joe	Jonnathon	Joseph	Juddson	Justinn	Kaiden
Joed	Jonnie	Josephe	Jude	Justino	Kaif
Joel	Jonny	Josephus	Judge	Justis	Kaiis
Joen	Jono	Josh	Judson	Justo	Kaikura
Joey	Jonte	Joshua	Juelz	Juston	Kail
Joffrey	Jonty	Joshuaa	Juha	Justus	Kaila
Johaan	Joop	Joshuah	Juke	Justyn	Kailas
Johan	Joosef	Joshwa	Jukka	Juvenal	Kaili
Johann	Joost	Josiah	Julen	Juwaan	Kaimana
Johannes	Jopie	Josias	Jules	Juwann	Kaimi
Johar	Joplin	Josidiah	Julian	Jye	Kain
John	Jor-el	Josilyn	Juliano	Jyler	Kaine
John-Paul	Jorah	Joss	Julien		Kaipo
Johnathan	Joram	Jossiah	Julienn	**K**	Kairi
Johnathon	Jordaan	Jossue	Julio		Kairos
Johnavan	Jordain	Josu	Julito	Kaamil	Kairu
Johnavon	Jordan	Josue	Julius	Kaapo	Kaiser
Johnn	Jordell	Jotham	Jullian	Kaarle	Kaison
Johnnathan	Jorden	Jothan	Jullien	Kaarlo	Kaito
Johnnathon	Jordence	Jouke	Jullius	Kaawa	Kaius
Johnnie	Jordi	Jourdain	July	Kabecka	Kaj
Johnny	Jordon	Jourdaine	Jumoke	Kabili	Kajetan

36

Kajika	Kana	Karsten	Kaycee	Keefer	Kellam
Kal-el	Kanaifu	Karston	Kayden	Keegan	Kellan
Kala	Kanan	Karter	Kaylor	Keelan	Kellen
Kalan	Kanapima	Kartik	Kayo	Keeley	Keller
Kalani	Kandoro	Kasabian	Kayode	Keelin	Kelley
Kalari	Kane	Kase	Kayonga	Keely	Kelli
Kalb	Kanelo	Kaseko	Kaysar	Keemeone	Kellsie
Kale	Kanga	Kasen	Kaysen	Keen	Kelly
Kaleb	Kanha	Kasey	Kayson	Keenan	Kelsea
Kaleeb	Kaniel	Kash	Kayvan	Keene	Kelsey
Kalei	Kanishka	Kasi	Kaywar	Keenen	Kelso
Kalel	Kannan	Kasim	Kaz	Keenon	Kelson
Kalem	Kannen	Kasimir	Kazi	Keeon	Keltie
Kalen	Kannon	Kason	Kazimierz	Keeran	Kelton
Kaleo	Kano	Kaspar	Kazmer	Kees	Kelven
Kaley	Kanoa	Kasper	Kazou	Keeshawn	Kelvhan
Kali	Kanoro	Kass	Kazuhito	Keeton	Kelvin
Kalida	Kansas	Kassidy	Kazuki	Keevan	Kelvis
Kalil	Kanye	Kassim	Kazuo	Keevin	Kelvyn
Kalin	Kaori	Katana	Kazutaka	Keeyon	Kelwin
Kaliq	Kapena	Katar	Kazuya	Kefir	Kelwyn
Kalkin	Kapil	Katashi	Kazuyuki	Keften	Kelyn
Kalle	Kapono	Kateb	Kea	Kegan	Keme
Kalleb	Karam	Katet	Keagan	Kehinde	Kemen
Kalman	Karan	Kathan	Keaghan	Kei	Kemp
Kalogeros	Karcsi	Katia	Keahi	Keifer	Kempton
Kaloosh	Kare	Kato	Keala	Keiffer	Kemuel
Kaltan	Kareem	Katriel	Kealan	Keiji	Ken
Kalum	Karel	Katsu	Kealii	Keiki	Ken'Ichi
Kalvin	Karen	Katsuo	Keallach	Keilah	Kenaan
Kalyan	Kari	Katsuro	Kealy	Keillan	Kenadie
Kam	Karif	Katsurou	Kean	Keir	Kenan
Kamal	Karik	Katungi	Keanan	Keiran	Kenaz
Kamali	Karim	Katyr	Keandre	Keisuke	Kenchiro
Kamari	Karin	Katzir	Keane	Keita	Kenchirou
Kamau	Karl	Kauai	Keani	Keitaro	Kendahl
Kamber	Karlens	Kaufman	Keannen	Keith	Kendal
Kamden	Karlheinz	Kauko	Keanu	Kek	Kendale
Kamdyn	Karlis	Kaushal	Kearn	Kekoa	Kendall
Kame	Karlitis	Kavan	Kearney	Keladry	Kendel
Kamea	Karlton	Kavanagh	Keary	Kelan	Kendi
Kameron	Karman	Kavanaugh	Keaton	Kelby	Kendis
Kameryn	Karmel	Kaveh	Keats	Keldan	Kendon
Kami	Karmi	Kaven	Keb	Kelden	Kendrell
Kamil	Karol	Kavi	Kedar	Keldon	Kendrew
Kamin	Karolek	Kavon	Kedem	Kele	Kendric
Kammeron	Karoly	Kawena	Kedric	Keletheryl	Kendrick
Kamran	Karr	Kay	Kedrick	Kelii	Kendrik
Kamron	Karsen	Kayan	Kedron	Kell	Kendrix
Kamryn	Karson	Kayce	Keefe	Kellagh	Kenelm

Kenji	Kernaghan	Khalfan	Kiet	Kippie	Knightley
Kenjiro	Kerouac	Khalid	Kieve	Kirabo	Knoll
Kenley	Kerr	Khalifa	Kiffen	Kiral	Knoton
Kenly	Kerrick	Khalil	Kiho	Kiran	Knox
Kenn	Kerrie	Khalil	Kiing	Kirby	Knud
Kennan	Kerrigan	Khalill	Kija	Kiri	Knut
Kennard	Kerry	Khaliq	Kijana	Kiril	Knute
Kenndrick	Kershet	Khallid	Kijani	Kirill	knute
Kennedy	Kerstan	Khallil	Kildare	Kirit	Ko
Kennelly	Kert	Khalon	Kile	Kirk	Koa
Kenner	Kervin	Khan	Kiley	Kirkan	Kobby
Kenneth	Kerwin	Khanh	Kilian	Kirkland	Kobe
Kenney	Kerwyn	Kharif	Killian	Kirkley	Kobi
Kennon	Kerym	Kharis	Kilydd	Kirklin	Koby
Kenny	Keryth	Khatar	Kim	Kirkwell	Koda
Kenric	Kesefehon	Khayrat	Kimball	Kirkwood	Kodey
Kenrick	Kesey	Khayri	Kimberly	Kiros	Kodi
Kenrik	Keshawn	Khayyam	Kimble	Kirsten	Kodiak
Kensey	Kesler	Khidell	Kimeya	Kirton	Kodie
Kenshin	Kesley	Khiiral	Kimn	Kishan	Kodjo
Kensington	Kester	Khilseith	Kimo	Kishi	Kody
Kensley	Kestrel	Khoi	Kimoni	Kismet	Koen
Kent	Ketan	Khoury	Kimotho	Kiss	Koenraad
Kenta	Ketill	Khristos	Kin	Kistna	Kofi
Kentaro	Keto	Khrystiyanr	Kincaid	Kit	Kohaku
Kentavious	Kettil	Khuong	Kindle	Kitchi	Kohana
Kenton	Kevan	Khuumal	Kindroth	Kitkun	Kohei
Kentrell	Keven	Khuyen	Kinfe	Kito	Kohen
Kentucky	Keveon	Khyrmn	King	Kitoko	Kohl
Kenward	Keverne	Kiaan	King Tut	Kitt	Koi
Kenway	Kevin	Kiah	Kingman	Kitto	Kojo
Kenya	Kevinn	Kian	Kingsley	Kivessin	Kolbjorn
Kenyatta	Kevion	Kiango	Kingston	Kiyohiko	Kolby
Kenyi	Kevis	Kianni	Kingswell	Kiyoshi	Kole
Kenyon	Kevon	Kiano	Kinion	Kiyuigh	Koleman
Kenzie	Kevork	Kiasax	Kinley	Kizzy	Kolichiyaw
Kenzo	Kevron	Kiba	Kinnard	Kjartan	Kolin
Keoki	Kevyn	Kibo	Kinnell	Kjell	Kollin
Keola	Key	Kick	Kinney	Klaasr	Kolt
Keon	Keyes	Kidd	Kinnon	Klaern	Kolten
Keondre	Keyne	Kiefer	Kinny	Klas	Koltin
Keoni	Keyon	Kieffer	Kinsella	Klaus	Kolton
Kepler	Keyonn	Kiel	Kinsey	Klay	Koltyn
Keran	Keyshawn	Kienan	Kinsley	Klayton	Kolvar
Kerem	Keyvan	Kier	Kinta	Klee	Kolya
Kerk	Kfir	Kieran	Kione	Klein	Konala
Kerman	Khaalid	Kierce	Klp	Klemens	Konane
Kermichi	Khadim	Kiernan	Kipling	Kleng	Kondo
Kermit	Khaled	Kieron	Kipp	Kliment	Kong
Kern	Khaleel	Kierron	Kippar	Knight	Konner

Konnor	Kristoff	Kymil	Laec	Landin	Lark
Konrad	Kristoffer	Kynan	Lael	Landis	Larkin
Konstancji	Kristofr	Kynaston	Laeroth	Lando	Larnell
Konstantin	Kristopher	KyndMryn	Laertes	Landon	Larongar
Konstantine	Krisztian	Kyne	Laestrygones	Landonn	Larrel
Kool	Kruz	Kynedyr	Lafarallin	Landry	Larrimore
Kopin	Krystupasr	Kynlas	Lafayette	Landyn	Larron
Koppel	Krzysztof	Kynon	Lafcadio	Lane	Larry
Kora	Krzysztofr	Kynton	Laidley	Laneetees	Lars
Korben	Kuckunniwi	Kynwal	Laik	Laney	Larue
Korbin	Kuirilr	Kynwyl	Lailoken	Lanford	Larz
Kordell	Kulon	Kyo	Lain	Lang	Lasalle
Koren	Kumar	Kyösti	Laine	Langdon	Lashawn
Koresh	Kumba	Kyosuke	Laird	Langer	Lashul
Korey	Kumi	Kyoto	Lais	Langford	Laszlo
Korian	Kunle	Kyou	Laiurenty	Langhorne	Lathai
Kornel	Kuornos	Kyran	Laius	Langley	Latham
Korrey	Kuper	Kyree	Lajos	Langston	Lathan
Kort	Kuro	Kyrell	Lake	Langundo	Lathlaeril
Korudon	Kuron	Kyrie	Lakeland	Langward	Lathrop
Kory	Kurou	Kyrillos	Laken	Langworth	Latif
Kosmosr	Kurt	Kyrillosr	Lakota	Lani	Latimer
Kosta	Kurtis	Kyrone	Lakshman	Lanier	Latinus
Kostya	Kuruk	Kyros	Lakyle	Lankston	Latrell
Kosuke	Kuskyn	Kyrtaar	Lalan	Lann	Laud
Kosumi	Kuthun	Kyson	Lalawethika	Lanndon	Laughlin
Kota	Kuval	Kywrkh	Lalla	Lanney	Launcelot
Kotori	Kwabena		Lalo	Lanny	Laurean
Koty	Kwahu	**L**	Lalor	Lansa	Lauren
Kouki	Kwame		Lam	Lansing	Laurence
Kourosh	Kwan	L'Angley	Lamaar	Lanston	Laurens
Kourtney	Kwanza	Laban	Lamar	Lanton	Laurent
Kouta	Kwasi	Labhrainn	Lamarcus	Lany	Laurente
Kovit	Kwatoko	Labhras	Lamarr	Lanza	Laurian
Kozue	Kwende	Labyrinth	Lambert	Lanzo	Laurie
Kraig	Kwint	Lacey	Lambi	Laochailan	Lauriston
Kramer	Kyan	Lach	Lamont	Laocoon	Lauritz
Kranich	Kyd	Lache	Lamruil	Laomedon	Lauro
Kratos	Kyden	Lachlan	Lancaster	Laosx	Lavan
Krikor	Kye	Lachlann	Lance	Lapidos	Lave
Kris	Kylan	Lachman	Lancel	Lapidoth	Lavender
Krischnan	Kylar	Lacrossc	Lancelin	Lapo	Laver
Krish	Kyle	Lacy	Lancelot	Lapu	Laverick
Krishna	Kyledyr	Ladarius	Land	Laramie	Laverne
Krispin	Kylemore	Ladbroc	Landan	Laran	Lavey
Krisstopher	Kylen	Ladd	Landdon	Larch	Lavi
Krister	Kyler	Laddie	Landen	Lardner	Lavonte
Kristian	Kyller	Ladell	Landenn	Laredo	Law
Kristof	Kylor	Ladislas	Lander	Laren	Lawford
Kristofer	Kymani	Ladon	Landers	Largo	Lawler

Lawley	Leif	Leslie	Lieven	Llarm	Lolonyo
Lawrence	Leigh	Lester	Light	Llassar	Lolovivi
Lawry	Leighton	Lethe	Liiam	Llawr	Loman
Lawson	Leith	Lev	Liko	Lleu	Lombard
Lawton	Lel	Levander	Lilo	Llevelys	Lon
Lawyer	Leland	Levant	Limon	Llew	Lonan
Layne	Lem	Leven	Linc	Llewellyn	Lonato
Layre	Leman	Leveret	Lincoln	Llewellenar	London
Laythan	Lemuel	Leverett	Lindberg	Llewellyn	Londyn
Layton	Len	Levey	Lindell	Llewelyn	Lonell
Lazar	Lenard	Levi	Lindeman	Lleyton	Long
Lazare	Lencho	Leviathan	Linden	Llombaerth	Longfellow
Lazaro	Lennan	Levii	Lindford	Lloyd	Lonnell
Lazarus	Lennard	Levin	Lindhurst	Lludd	Lonnie
Lazer	Lennie	Leviticus	Lindley	Llundein	Lonny
Lazlo	Lenno	Levka	Lindon	Llwybyr	Lonzo
Lazzaro	Lennon	Levon	Lindsay	Llwyd	Lootah
Leaf	Lennox	Levron	Lindsey	Llwydeu	Lorand
Leal	Lenny	Levy	Line	Llwyr	Lorant
Leander	Leno	Lew	Linh	Llyn	Lorcan
Leandre	Leo	Lewellyn	Link	Llyr	Lord
Leandrew	Leocadie	Lewi	Linley	Llyweilun	Lore
Leandro	Leod	Lewin	Linn	Llywelyn	Loren
Leandros	Leodegan	Lewis	Linnaeus	Loba	Lorence
Lear	Leodegrance	Lex	Lino	Lobo	Lorenz
Leary	Leodegraunce	Lexer	Lintang	Loc	Lorenzo
Leathan	Leojym	Lexington	Linton	Loch	Lorimer
Leavitt	Leomaris	Lexis	Linus	Lochlainn	Lorin
Leb	Leon	Lexus	Linwood	Lochlan	Loring
Lebeau	Leonard	Leyti	Lion	Lochlann	Lorne
Lebron	Leonardo	Lezane	Lionel	Locke	Lornell
Lebrun	Leonce	Lhoris	Lionell	Lockhart	Lorrenzo
Lech	Leone	Li	Lior	Lockwood	Lorrimer
Lee	Leonel	Lia	Lippio	Lodge	Lorry
Leeo	Leonell	Liam	Liron	Lodovico	Lorsan
Leeon	Leonid	Liamm	Lisandro	Lodur	Lot
Leeroy	Leonidas	Liander	Lise	Loe	Lotan
Leetov	Leonide	Liandro	Lisle	Loeb	Lotem
Leevi	Leonides	Liang	Lissandro	Loew	Lothair
Leevon	Leonitus	Lianthorn	Lister	Loewy	Lothar
Lefty	Leonore	Liav	Lito	Loften	Lotus
Legend	Leontios	Liberato	Little	Logan	Lou
Legget	Leopold	Liberio	Litton	Logen	Loudon
Leggett	Leopoldo	Liberty	Liuz	Loggan	Loughlin
Legolas	Lerato	Liborio	Lively	Loic	Louie
Legrand	Leroi	Lichas	Livingston	Lok	Louis
Lehana	Leron	Lidio	Liviu	Lokesh	Loukas
Lehman	Leroux	Lidon	Liwanu	Loki	Louvain
Leib	Leroy	Lidskjalf	Llacheu	Lokni	Louvel
Leicester	Les	Liev	Llara	Lolek	Love

Lovell	Luken	Lyon	Machi	Maelwys	Maimon
Lovender	Lukka	Lyonechka	Machk	Maemi	Maimun
Lowe	Lukkas	Lyonya	Machum	Maeraddyth	Mainchin
Lowell	Lukman	Lyova	Mack	Maeral	Maine
Lowman	Lukyan	Lyre	Mackenzie	Maeron	Mairtin
Lowry	Lulani	Lyric	MacKenzie	Maeryn	Maison
Loxias	Lun	Lysander	Mackinac	Magal	Maitho
Loyal	Lunaire	Lysanthir	Mackinley	Magan	Maitland
Luano	Lundie	Lyting	MacKinley	Magar	Maj
Lubomir	Lundy	Lytton	Macklin	Magaska	Majed
Luboslaw	Lunn	Lyuben	Macklyn	Magda	Majesty
Luc	Luol		Mackson	Maged	Majid
Luca	Luqman	**M**	MacLaren	Magee	Major
Lucan	Luthais		Maclean	Maggio	Makai
Lucas	Luthando	Maalik	Macmahon	Magic	Makaio
Lucca	Luther	Maanav	Macmurray	Magnar	Makalo
Luccas	Luukas	Maarten	MacNab	Magni	Makan
Lucciano	Luvon	Mablevi	Macniel	Magnild	Makani
Luce	Lux	Mabon	Macon	Magnum	Makari
Lucero	Luxovious	Mabry	Maconaquea	Magnus	Makarios
Lucian	Luz	Mabsant	MacPherson	Maguire	Makeiah
Luciano	Ly	Mac	Macrae	Magus	Makena
Lucien	Lyaksandro	Macadam	Macsen	Mahak	Makhi
Lucifer	Lyall	Macall	Macy	Mahari	Makin
Lucila	Lyam	Macallister	Madaleno	Mahaskah	Makis
Lucilius	Lyari	Macardle	Madan	Mahatma	Makisig
Lucio	Lycaon	Macario	Madawc	Mahavira	Makkapitew
Lucius	Lycomedes	Macarius	Madawg	Mahdi	Maklolm
Lucky	Lycurgus	Macarthur	Madden	Mahendra	Makolm
Lucretius	Lycus	Macaulay	Madison	Maher	Makoto
Lucus	Lydell	Macauley	Maddison	Mahesh	Makram
Ludano	Lydon	Macbeth	Maddoc	Mahfuz	Maks
Ludlow	Lyel	Macbride	Maddock	Mahieu	Maksim
Ludo	Lyklor	Maccabee	Maddockson	Mahir	Maksimillian
Ludoslaw	Lyle	Maccaulay	Maddocson	Mahkah	Maksym
Ludovic	Lyman	Maccoy	Maddog	Mahlon	Maksymilian
Ludvik	Lynceus	Macdonald	Maddox	Mahmood	Makya
Ludwig	Lynch	Macdougal	Madelon	Mahmoud	Mal
Ludwik	Lyndal	Mace	Madesio	Mahmud	Malachi
Lufti	Lynde	Macedonio	Madigan	Mahomet	Malachy
Lug	Lynden	Maceo	Madison	Mahon	Maladec
Lughaidh	Lyndon	Macerio	Madoc	Mahpee	Maladcck
Luigi	Lyndsey	Macfarlane	Madog	Mai	Maladek
Luirlan	Lynford	MacGillivray	Madrid	Maichail	Malak
Luis	Lynk	Macgowan	Mads	Maiele	Malakai
Lujan	Lynley	MacGregor	Madu	Maik	Malaki
Luka	Lynn	Macgregor	Mael	Mailer	Malakii
Lukas	Lynne	Machakw	Maeleachlainn	Mailhairer	Malcolm
Lukasz	Lynton	Machau	Maelgwyn	Maille	Malcom
Luke	Lynx	Machenry	Maelisa	Maillol	Malden

Malek	Manjit	Marcell	Marlevaur	Marv	Mathias
Maleko	Manju	Marcellin	Marley	Marvel	Mathieu
Malgath	Mankato	Marcellino	Marlin	Marvell	Mathis
Maliik	Manley	Marcello	Marlo	Marven	Matias
Malik	Mann	Marcellus	Marlon	Marvin	Matin
Malikk	Mannan	Marcelo	Marlow	Marwan	Matisse
Malin	Manneville	Marcely	Marlowe	Marwood	Mato
Maliq	Mannheim	March	Marlyssa	Maryland	Matoskah
Malise	Mannie	Marcian	Marmaduke	Marylu	Matrim
Malki	Manning	Marciano	Marmion	Masaru	Matro
Mallaki	Mannix	Marcin	Marnin	Masashi	Mats
Malleville	Mannuss	Marcinek	Marnix	Masefield	Matsu
Mallik	Manny	Marcio	Maro	Mashaka	Matt
Mallolwch	Mano	Marco	Marom	Masichuvio	Mattanyah
Mallory	Manoach	Marcos	Marq	Masih	Mattathias
Mallow	Manolito	Marcus	Marque	Maska	Matteo
Malloy	Manolo	Marcuss	Marques	Maslin	Matteus
Malo	Mansel	Mardeiym	Marquette	Maso	Matthew
Malone	Mansfield	Mardel	Marquez	Mason	Matthias
Maloney	Mansoor	Marden	Marquis	Masood	Matthieu
Malus	Mansour	Mardon	Marquise	Masos	Matthijs
Malvin	Mansur	Mare	Marquiss	Masoud	Mattia
Malyn	Mantel	Marek	Marr	Massachusetts	Mattias
Maminnic	Manton	Mareo	Marrim	Massai	Mattie
Mamun	Mantotohpa	Mariam	Marriner	Masselin	Mattijs
Mana	Manu	Marian	Marrio	Massey	Mattityahu
Manal	Manuel	Mariano	Marrk	Massika	Mattox
Manas	Manuelo	Mariatu	Mars	Massimo	Mattthew
Manasseh	Manus	Maribelle	Marsden	Masson	Matty
Manasses	Manvel	Marikoth	Marsh	Maston	Matunaagd
Manawydan	Manvil	Marin	Marshal	Masud	Matvey
Mance	Manville	Marinel	Marshall	Mat	Matwau
Manchester	Manzie	Marino	Marshawn	Matai	Matyas
Mancuso	Manzo	Mario	Marston	Matan	Matysh
Mandan	Manzu	Marion	Martainn	Mataniah	Matz
Mandar	Maolmin	Marius	Martel	Matar	Matzliach
Mandek	Maolmuire	Marji	Martell	Matchitehew	Maughold
Mandel	Maolruadhan	Mark	Martelli	Matchitisiw	Mauli
Mandela	Maonaigh	Marka	Marten	Mate	Maur
Mandell	Maovesa	Markell	Martez	Mateja	Maureo
Mandeville	Maoz	Markey	Martijn	Mateo	Maurice
Mandla	Mar	Markham	Martin	Mateus	Mauricio
Mando	Maralyn	Markk	Martinez	Mateusz	Maurilio
Mane	Maram	Markku	Martinien	Math	Maurio
Manelin	Marc	Markkus	Martino	Mathe	Maurizio
Manfred	Marcario	Marko	Martinus	Mather	Mauro
Manfried	Marcas	Markov	Martirio	Matheus	Maurus
Manfrit	Marceau	Markus	Marton	Mathew	Maury
Mani	Marcel	Marland	Marty	Mathews	Maurycy
Manis	Marcelino	Marlas	Martyn	Mathhew	Mauty

42

Maverick	McKile	Melburn	Meridith	Michael	Mikkel
Mavrick	Mckinley	Melbyrne	Meris	Michaiah	Mikko
Mawrth	McKinley	Melchior	Merith	Michail	Miklos
Max	McLovin	Melchisedek	Merivale	Michal	Miko
Maxen	Mead	Melchoir	Merkaba	Micheal	Mikolai
Maxence	Meade	Meldon	Merla	Micheál	Mikolaj
Maxfield	Meadhra	Meldrick	Merle	Micheil	Mikolas
Maxim	Meara	Mele	Merlin	Michel	Mil
Maxime	Mecca	Melech	Merlion	Michelangelo	Milad
Maximilian	Medad	Melesio	Merlow	Michele	Milagro
Maximiliano	Medan	Melicertes	Merlyn	Michi	Milan
Maximillian	Medford	Melker	Meron	Michiaki	Miland
Maximino	Medric	Melky	Merric	Michigan	Milandu
Maximo	Medus	Mellen	Merrick	Michio	Milap
Maximos	Medwin	Melor	Merrill	Michon	Milbank
Maximus	Medwyn	Melrone	Merritt	Mick	Milburn
Maxon	Medyr	Melville	Mersey	Mickel	Milek
Maxton	Meegwin	Melvin	Merton	Mickey	Milen
Maxwell	Mees	Melvon	Merv	Mico	Miles
Maxxim	Meged	Melvyn	Mervin	Micol	Milford
Maxximus	Megedagik	Memengwa	Mervyn	Midas	Milintica
Maxy	Meghdad	Memphis	Merwin	Middleton	Millan
Mayer	Mego	Menachem	Merwyn	Midhat	Millard
Mayes	Meguinis	Menashe	Meryl	Midian	Millen
Mayfield	Mehdi	Menassah	Meryle	Midnight	Miller
Mayhew	Mehmood	Menawa	Meshach	Mies	Mills
Mayir	Mehmud	Mendel	Meshar	Migdal	Milne
Maynard	Mehran	Mendie	Messiah	Migisi	Milo
Mayne	Mehrdad	Menefer	Messina	Miguel	Milos
Maynor	Meilseoir	Menelaus	Metcalf	Mihaly	Miloslav
Mayo	Meilyg	Meng	Meteor	Mihammad	Milt
Mayson	Meilyr	Menoeceus	Methild	Mihangel	Milton
Mazablaska	Meinhard	Mensonsea	Methodios	Mihangyl	Mimir
Mazatl	Meinke	Mentari	Methuselah	Miichael	Min
Mazin	Meino	Mentor	Meturato	Miikka	Minal
Mazor	Meinrad	Menw	Meurig	Miirphys	Mincho
Mcarthur	Meinyard	Menzies	Meyer	Mijndert	Miner
Mccabe	Meir	Meo	Meztli	Mika	Ming
McCai	Meitar	Mer	Mhaenal	Mikael	Ming Yue
Mccanna	Mekaisto	Merc	Mhina	Mikaia	Mingan
Mccoy	Mekhi	Mercator	Mi'tilarro	Mikaili	Mingus
Mccrea	Mel	Merce	Miach	Mikasi	Minh
Mcdermott	Melampus	Mercer	Mica	Mike	Minnesota
Mcenroe	Melancton	Mercher	Micah	Mikee	Minninnewah
Mcewan	Melandrach	Mercury	Micaiah	Mikel	Minor
McIntyre	Melanion	Meredith	Micajah	Mikey	Minoru
McKale	Melanippus	Meredydd	Micchael	Mikhail	Minos
Mckenna	Melanthius	Merek	Micha	Mikhalis	Minowa
McKenna	Melborn	Merellien	Michaael	Mikhos	Minster
McKenzie	Melbourne	Meridian	Michaeel	Miki	Mint

Minze	Modred	Montagor	Morio	Mubin	Myrddin
Mio	Moe	Montague	Moritz	Mufaddal	Myrick
Miquel	Moesen	Montaigu	Moriz	Muga	Myriil
Miracle	Moeshe	Montaine	Morland	Mugisa	Myrin
Mirage	Mogue	Montana	Morley	Muhammad	Myron
Miraj	Mohajit	Montaro	Moroccan	Muhammed	Mythanthar
Mirin	Mohamed	Montay	Morocco	Muhsin	
Miró	Mohammad	Monte	Morogh	Muhsina	**N**
Miron	Mohammed	Montee	Morpheus	Muir	
Miroslav	Mohan	Montego	Morrey	Muircheartaigh	Naal
Mirren	Mohandas	Montel	Morrie	Muireadhach	Naalnish
Mirthal	Mohave	Montell	Morrigan	Mukhtar	Naalyehe
Mirza	Mohawk	Montenegro	Morris	Mukki	Naaman
Misae	Mohegan	Montes	Morrisey	Mukonry	Naasir
Misael	Mohsen	Montez	Morrison	Mulcahy	Nab
Mischa	Moise	Montezuma	Morrissey	Muller	Nabil
Misha	Moises	Montgomery	Morrow	Mulligan	Nachman
Mishael	Moishe	Montreal	Morse	Muna	Nachmanke
Mishal	Moisses	Montrel	Mort	Muncel	Nacho
Mishe	Mojag	Montrell	Morten	Munchin	Nachshon
Mishenka	Mojave	Montrelle	Morthil	Mundy	Nachton
Mishka	Mojil	Monty	Morthwyl	Mungo	Nachum
Misi	Mokatavatah	Moody	Mortimer	Muni	Nacio
Miska	Moke	Moon	Morton	Munin	Nadav
Mississippi	Moketoveto	Moor	Morty	Munir	Nadia
Missouri	Moki	Moore	Morvan	Munro	Nadim
Mistral	Mokovaoto	Mopsus	Morven	Muntasir	Nadir
Misu	Molan	Morain	Morvran	Muraco	Nadiv
Mitali	Molimo	Moral	Mosaed	Murad	Naeem
Mitch	Molli	Moran	Mose	Murchadh	Naertho
Mitchel	Molloy	Morandi	Moseph	Murdock	Naeryndam
Mitchell	Molonym	Morathi	Moses	Muriel	Naftali
Mitford	Molostroi	Morcan	Moshe	Murphy	Naftalie
Mith	Momchil	Morcar	Mosheh	Murray	Nagel
Mitra	Momus	Mordecai	Mosi	Murron	Nagelfar
Mitsu	Mona	Mordechai	Moss	Murrow	Naggar
Mitt	Monaco	Mordwywr	Mosses	Murry	Nagid
Mizell	Monahan	More	Mostafa	Murtada	Nagisa
Mizu	Monchonsia	Moreland	Mostyn	Murtaugh	Nahcomence
Mjolnir	Monckton	Moreley	Motavato	Murtaza	Nahele
Mladen	Monet	Morell	Motega	Musoke	Nahiossi
Mlartlar	Mongo	Moren	Motka	Mustafa	Nahir
Mo	Mongwau	Morey	Motke	Muunokhoi	Nahma
Moab	Monico	Morgan	Mouna	Mychajlo	Nahuatl
Mobley	Monkaushka	Morgannwg	Mowanza	Mycroft	Nahuel
Moby	Monone	Morgen	Mowgli	Myer	Nahum
Mochan	Monroe	Mori	Mowway	Mykelti	Naif
Mochni	Mons	Moriarty	Mozart	Mykhaltso	Nail
Modesto	Montae	Moricz	Mu	Mylan	Naim
Modi	Montagew	Moriel	Muata	Myles	Nairi

44

Nairn	Nardual	Naveed	Neilson	Newat	Nicol
Nairne	Naren	Naveen	Neka	Newbold	Nicola
Nairobi	Naresh	Navid	Nelaeryn	Newbury	Nicolaas
Naiser	Nari	Navigator	Neldor	Newcomb	Nicolai
Naji	Nariman	Navin	Nelek	Newell	Nicolao
Najib	Nario	Naviyd	Neleus	Newlyn	Nicolas
Najinca	Narius	Navon	Nelius	Newland	Nicolaus
Nakia	Narkis	Navy	Nelly	Newlin	Nicoli
Nakos	Naruto	Naw	Nelo	Newlyn	Nicollas
Nakotah	Narve	Nawat	Nels	Newman	Nicolo
Nakula	Narvel	Nawkaw	Nelson	Newport	Nicomedes
Nalani	Nash	Nawwar	Nelton	Newt	Nida
Naldo	Nasha	Nayan	Nemesio	Newton	Niel
Nalin	Nashua	Nayati	Nemo	Newyddllyn	Niels
Nalo	Nasiir	Nayef	Nemos	Neymar	Nieven
Nam	Nasim	Nayland	Nen	Nezer	Nigan
Namaka	Nasir	Naylor	Neo	Nguyen	Nigel
Naman	Nasli	Nazaire	Neomonni	Nhamashal	Nigell
Namas	Nasmith	Nazareth	Neptune	Niabi	Night
Name	Nasser	Nazario	Nequiel	Niall	Nightshade
Namid	Nastas	Nazih	Ner	Niatohsa	Niguel
Namir	Nat	Neacal	Nereus	Niaz	Niichaad
Nana	Natal	Neakail	Nergui	Nibal	Nik
Nando	Natalio	Neal	Neriah	Nibaw	Nike
Nann	Natan	Neale	Nero	Nicabar	Nikeiza
Nanne	Natanael	Neall	Neron	Nicandro	Nikhil
Nansen	Natanel	Nealon	Nerth	Nicanor	Niki
Nantai	Natania	Neander	Nerthach	Nicasio	Nikifor
Naoki	Nataniel	Neason	Neruda	Niccolas	Nikita
Naolin	Nate	Neb	Nesbit	Niccolo	Nikiti
Naomhan	Nathair	Nebo	Ness	Nichol	Nikki
Naor	Nathan	Nebraska	Nessan	Nichola	Nikko
Naoya	Nathanael	Nebula	Nesterin	Nicholaas	Nikkolai
Napayshni	Nathanial	Necalli	Nesto	Nicholai	Nikkos
Napeu	Nathaniel	Nechemiah	Nestor	Nicholas	Niklas
Napezi	Nathaniell	Nechemya	Nethanel	Nicholaus	Niklaus
Naphtali	Nathann	Nechtan	Neto	Nicholes	Niko
Napier	Nathen	Neckarios	Netra	Nichollas	Nikodem
Napoleon	Nathrach	Nectarios	Netro	Nichols	Nikola
Napowsa	Nathraichean	Ned	Neued	Nicholson	Nikolai
Naquan	Natine	Neel	Neuveville	Nicias	Nikolajis
Narain	Natividad	Neely	Nevada	Nick	Nikolas
Naranbaatar	Natsu	Nef	Nevan	Nicklaus	Nikolaus
Narayan	Natthan	Negasi	Nevarth	Nickleby	Nikolos
Narbeth	Nature	Nehemiah	Neville	Nickolai	Nikos
Narcisco	Naughton	Nehru	Nevin	Nickolas	Nikostratos
Narcisse	Naum	Neifion	Nevins	Nickson	Nila
Narcissus	Nauplius	Neil	Nevio	Nicky	Nilax
Nard	Navarone	Neilan	Nevyn	Nico	Nile
Nardo	Navarro	Neill	New	Nicodemus	Niles

45

Nili	Nobu	Notchimine	O'Grady	Odo	Olaurae
Nilo	Nobuhide	Notin	O'Hara	Odolf	Ole
Nilos	Noburu	Notus	O'Keefe	Odran	Oleg
Nils	Nobuyuki	Noud	O'Neal	Odysseus	Oles
Nilsen	Noda	Nouel	O'Reilly	Oedipus	Olexei
Nilsson	Nodin	Nour	O'Shea	Oenel	Olezka
Nima	Noe	Nouvel	O'Sullivan	Oeneus	Olimpio
Nimai	Noel	Nova	Oacenth	Oengus	Olin
Nimat	Noell	Novak	Oachim	Oenomaus	Olindo
Nimrod	Noelle	November	Oak	Ofek	Oliver
Nin	Nogah	Novena	Oakes	Ofer	Oliverio
Nindrol	Nohea	Nowles	Oakley	Ofir	Oliverios
Ning	Noire	Nox	Oan	Ofra	Olivier
Ninian	Nolan	Noy	Oba	Ofydd	Ollie
Nino	Noland	Noyce	Obadiah	Ogaleesha	Olliver
Ninthalor	Nolen	Nremyn	Obadias	Ogden	Olof
Nir	Nollan	Nuhad	Obama	Ogen	Olsen
Niran	Nollie	Nukpana	Obed	Ogilhinn	Olson
Nirav	Nolyn	Numair	Obediah	Ogilvie	Olwydd
Nirel	Nonnie	Nuncio	Obelix	Ogilvy	Olympos
Nishan	Noon	Nur	Oberon	Ogima	Oma
Nissan	Noor	Nuren	Obert	Ogun	Omanand
Nissim	Nootau	Nuri	Obi	Ohad	Omar
Nissyen	Nopos	Nuriel	Obiareus	Ohan	Omari
Nisus	Norbert	Nuru	Obrien	Ohanko	Omarion
Nitesh	Norberto	Nuvian	Obsidian	Ohanzee	Omarr
Nitis	Norcross	Nyack	Occhave	Ohara	Omawnakw
Nitish	Noreis	Nyako	Ocean	Ohcumgache	Omeet
Nitzan	Norfolk	Nye	Oceanus	Ohio	Omega
Nitzchi	Nori	Nykko	Ocheckka	Ohitekah	Omeo
Niv	Norice	Nyle	Ocnus	Ohmbryn	Omer
Niven	Norm	Nyles	Octave	Ohtli	Omet
Nixen	Norman	Nylian	Octavian	Oidhche	Ometaway
Nixkamich	Normand	Nym	Octavio	Oighrig	Ommar
Nixon	Normando	Nynnyaw	Octavious	Oisin	Omri
Niyol	Normandy	Nyoka	Octavius	Oistin	On
Nizar	Norris	Nyree	October	Ojai	Onan
Njal	North	Nyvorlas	Ocunnowhurst	Ojas	Onas
Njord	Northcliff		Oda	Okal	Oncith
Njorthrbiartr	Northrop	O	Odakota	Okapi	Ondre
Nlossae	Norton		Odanodan	Oke	Ondrea
Noach	Norval	O'Brian	Oded	Okello	Ondyaw
Noadiah	Norville	O'Brien	Odell	Okena	Onfroi
Noah	Norvin	O'Callahan	Odgar	Okhmhaka	ONille
Noahh	Norvyn	O'Casey	Odhran	Oklahoma	Onni
Noam	Norward	O'Connor	Odilio	Okoth	Onofre
Noapeh	Norwell	O'Donnell	Odilo	Ol	Onofredo
Noaz	Norwood	O'Donovan	Odin	Ola	Onofrio
Noble	Nosh	O'Fallon	Odion	Olaf	Onslow
Noboru	Noshi		Odissan	Olan	Ontario

Onvyr	Ornette	Osmond	Oxide	Pagiel	Parc
Ony	Ornice	Osred	Oxley	Pahana	Pardes
Onyx	Orno	Osric	Oxton	Pahkakino	Parees
Ooyu	Ornthalas	Osrid	Oya	Pahukumaa	Paresh
Ophion	Oro	Ossian	Oyintsa	Paidi	Parfait
Ophir	Oron	Ossie	Oz	Paien	Parham
Or	Orpheus	Ossin	Ozer	Paige	Paris
Oracle	Orran	Osten	Ozi	Paine	Parish
Oral	Orrel	Osvaldo	Ozias	Painter	Park
Oran	Orren	Oswald	Ozni	Paisley	Parke
Orane	Orrick	Oswaldo	Ozur	Paitalyi	Parker
Oratilwe	Orrin	Oswallt	Ozuru	Pal	Parkin
Orazio	Orsen	Oswin	Ozzi	Palace	Parkins
Orde	Orsin	Otaehryn	Ozzie	Paladin	Parlan
Ordell	Orsino	Otaktay	Ozzy	Paladio	Parley
Orel	Orson	Othello		Palaemon	Parmenio
Orell	Ortega	Othman	**P**	Palamedes	Parnel
Oren	Orthros	Othniel		Palani	Parnell
Orenthal	Orton	Othorion	P'Adraic	Palash	Parr
Orestes	Orval	Otieno	Paavo	Palban	Parren
Oreta	Orvelle	Otilio	Pabiyan	Palben	Parrish
Orev	Orvil	Otis	Pablo	Palermo	Parry
Orfeo	Orville	Otniel	Pace	Paley	Parson
Orford	Orvin	Otoahhastis	Pacey	Palila	Parsons
Ori	Orym	Otoahnacto	Pacho	Palin	Parthalan
Oriel	Osage	Otos	Pachua	Pallas	Parthenios
Orien	Osama	Ottavio	Paciano	Pallaton	Parton
Orik	Osamu	Ottfried	Pacific	Palmer	Parvaiz
Orin	Osaze	Otto	Pacifico	Palomo	Parzifal
Oringo	Osbaldo	Otus	Packard	Paltel	Pascal
Oriol	Osbert	Ouray	Paco	Palti	Pascha
Oriole	Osborn	Ourson	Pacome	Paltiel	Pascoe
Orion	Osborne	Outacite	Pacorro	Pan	Pascual
Oris	Osbourne	Ovadia	Paddington	Panagiotis	Pasha
Orist	Oscar	Ovadiah	Paddy	Panas	Pashenka
Orlan	Osceola	Ovadya	Paden	Pancho	Pasqual
Orland	Oscosh	Ove	Padget	Pancratius	Pasquale
Orlando	Osei	Oved	Padgett	Pannoowau	Pastor
Orleans	Osgood	Overton	Padraic	Panos	Pat
Orlin	Osheen	Ovid	Padraig	Pantelcimon	Patamon
Orlondo	Osher	Ovidio	Pádraig	Panther	Patch
Orlpar	Osias	Owain	Padriac	Pany	Paterson
Orly	Osier	Owein	Padric	Panya	Patli
Orman	Osip	Owen	Padrig	Paolo	Paton
Ormand	Osiris	Owenn	Padruig	Papandrou	Patric
Ormando	Oskar	Owethu	Paeral	Paquito	Patrice
Ormond	Oslarelar	Owin	Paeris	Param	Patricio
Ormondo	Oslo	Owyn	Pagan	Paramesh	Patrick
Orn	Osman	Owynn	Page	Paras	Patrido
Orndacil	Osmar	Oxford	Paget	Paratyl	

Patrin	Peanut	Pepe	Petrelis	Phorcys	Piran
Patrizio	Pearce	Pepijn	Petrica	Phraan	Pirate
Patroclus	Pedahel	Pepillo	Petrini	Phrixus	Pirithous
Patryk	Peder	Pepin	Petros	Phuc	Piroj
Patsy	Pedr	Pepper	Petrov	Phuoc	Pirphal
Patten	Pedro	Pepperell	Petter	Phyllon	Pirro
Patterson	Peel	Peppin	Petuel	Phylo	Pisces
Patton	Peer	Peppino	Petya	Phyre	Pistol
Pattrick	Peerless	Per	Peverell	Piano	Pitney
Patty	Peers	Perceval	Peyton	Piapot	Pitt
Patwin	Peeta	Percival	Phaendar	Piav	Pittheus
Patxi	Pegalesharro	Percy	Phaethon	Picabia	Pius
Pauel	Pegasus	Perdana	Phantasos	Picard	Pizi
Paul	Pegeen	Perdido	Phaon	Picasso	Placido
Paulin	Pei	Peredur	Pharaoh	Piccolo	Plamen
Paulino	Peirce	Peregrine	Pharell	Pickford	Plantagenet
Paull	Peissawg	Peretz	Pharom	Picton	Plat
Paulo	Pekelo	Perez	Phelan	Pier	Plato
Paulos	Pelagios	Perfecto	Phelix	Pierce	Platon
Pavan	Pele	Pericles	Phelps	Pierluigi	Platt
Pavel	Peleg	Perico	Phemius	Piero	Plaxico
Pavlpv	Peleh	Perkin	Pherson	Pierpont	Plenty
Pavlik	Peleus	Perl	Phil	Pierre	Pleufan
Pavlo	Pelham	Pernell	Philadelphia	Pierrepont	Plexippus
Pavlos	Peli	Pero	Philander	Pierro	Plummer
Pavlusha	Pelias	Perren	Philbert	Piers	Pluto
Pavlushka	Pell	Perrin	Philemon	Pierson	Plutus
Pavlya	Pelle	Perry	Philihert	Piet	Plys
Pawel	Pellegrino	Perryn	Philip	Pieter	Po
Pawelek	Pelli	Perseus	Philipp	Pietr	Pochanaw
Pawl	Pello	Persia	Philippe	Pietrek	Poe
Pawnee	Pelops	Persius	Phill	Pietro	Poet
Pax	Pelton	Pert	Phillip	Pike	Pollux
Paxon	Pemberley	Perth	Phillipe	Pili	Pol
Paxton	Pembroke	Peru	Phillipp	Pilib	Poldi
Payat	Pemota	Pervis	Philo	Pillan	Pollard
Payatt	Pemton	Pesach	Philoctetes	Pilot	Pollock
Payden	Penda	Pesah	Philomena	Pim	Pollux
Payne	Pendle	Peso	Philomon	Pinchas	Polo
Pays	Pendleton	Pessach	Philosophy	Pine	Polydamas
Payson	Penha	Pete	Phinean	Ping	Polymestor
Paytah	Penllyn	Petenka	Phineas	Pino	Pom
Payton	Penley	Peter	Phineus	Pio	Pomeroy
Paz	Penn	Peterke	Phinnaeus	Piotr	Pommelraie
Pazel	Pennsylvania	Peterson	Phipps	Pip	Pompeo
Peabody	Penrod	Peteul	Phlegethon	Piper	Pompey
Peace	Penrose	Petey	Phoebus	Piperel	Ponce
Peadair	Pentheus	Petiri	Phoenix	Pippin	Pons
Peak	Penvro	Petit	Phomello	Pippino	Ponti
Peale	Pepa	Peton	Phong	Pippo	Pontifex

Ponto
Pontus
Pooh
Pope
Popo
Poppy
Porat
Porfirio
Porfiro
Poriel
Porsche
Porter
Porteur
Porthos
Portier
Portland
Poseanye
Poseidon
Posh
Poshita
Potter
Pouria
Povitamun
Poviyemo
Powa
Powasheek
Powell
Power
Powers
Powhatan
Powwaw
Pradeep
Prairie
Pranav
Pranet
Pratap
Pratt
Pravar
Pravat
Pravin
Praxis
Preben
Preece
Prem
Prentice
Preruet
Prescott
Presley
Press
Preston

Prewitt
Priam
Priapus
Price
Priel
Priest
Primeiro
Primo
Primus
Prince
Princeton
Prior
Priour
Prisco
Pritam
Probert
Procopio
Procrustes
Proctor
Prokhor
Prokopios
Prometheus
Prophyrios
Prosper
Prosperity
Prospero
Protesilaus
Proteus
Proust
Proverb
Provo
Prudencio
Pruet
Pruie
Pruitt
Pryce
Pryderi
Prydwen
Pryor
Prys
Prysm
Przemek
Przemo
Przemyslaw
Psalm
Psamtic
Ptolemy
Puck
Pueblo
Puma

Purtham
Purvis
Pushmataha
Putnam
Puw
Pwyll
Pygmalion
Pyotr
Pyralis
Pyramid
Pyramus
Pyrder
Pyrravym
Pyrs
Pywaln

Q

Qabil
Qadan
Qadar
Qadim
Qadir
Qaletaqa
Qamar
Qasim
Qays
Qiao
Qildor
Qimat
Qing Yuan
Qismat
Qochata
Quadarius
Quade
Quaid
Quain
Quana
Quanah
Quang
Quanmaine
Quant
Quantavius
Quany
Quarrie
Quarry
Quartz
Quashawn

Quasim
Quay
Quebec
Quenby
Quennel
Quennell
Quent
Quentin
Quenton
Quentrell
Queran
Querijn
Quesnel
Quest
Quico
Quigley
Quill
Quillan
Quillen
Quiller
Quilliam
Quillon
Quimby
Quin
Quince
Quincey
Quincy
Quinlan
Quinn
Quinncy
Quinnell
Quinney
Quinntin
Quinnton
Quint
Quintas
Quintavius
Quinten
Quintero
Quintin
Quinto
Quinton
Quintrell
Quintus
Quique
Quiqui
Quirin
Quirinal
Quirino
Quirt

Quirtsquip
Quito
Quixley
Quixote
Quoba
Quon
Qusay
Quynn
Qwin

R

R'phael
Raahul
Raanan
Rabbi
Rabi
Rabia
Race
Racer
Racham
Rachamim
Rad
Radames
Radbert
Radburn
Radcliff
Radek
Radford
Radimir
Radko
Radley
Radnor
Radorm
Radoslaw
Radwan
Rae
Raeburn
Raed
Raeranthur
Rafael
Rafaele
Rafaello
Rafal
Rafe
Rafer
Raffael
Raffaello
Rafferty
Rafi

Rafiki
Rafiq
Raghib
Raghnall
Ragnar
Ragnarok
Ragnor
Rahat
Raheem
Rahim
Rahul
Rai
Raibyr
Raidan
Raiden
Raidon
Raighne
Raimi
Raimond
Raimondo
Raimundo
Rain
Rainart
Raine
Rainer
Raines
Rainger
Rainier
Rais
Raith
Raj
Rajabu
Rajah
Rajan
Rajesh
Raji
Rajiv
Rajmund
Rajnish
Rakin
Raktim
Ralcigh
Ralikanthae
Rally
Ralnor
Ralph
Ralphie
Ralston
Ram
Rama

Raman	Rashadd	Raynor	Reiner	Reuhen	Rhys
Ramanan	Rashard	Rayvon	Reinier	Reule	Rhyson
Rambo	Rashaun	Raz	Reis	Reuven	Rhythm
Rami	Rashawn	Raziel	Rekker	Reve	Riad
Ramirez	Rasheed	Razo	Reluraun	Revelin	Riagan
Ramiro	Rashid	Read	Reluvethel	Rex	Riah
Ramon	Rashidi	Reade	Rem	Rexford	Rian
Ramond	Rasim	Reading	Rembrandt	Rexton	Riaz
Ramone	Rasmus	Reagan	Remedio	Rexx	Ric
Ramsay	Rastus	Reason	Remedy	Rey	Ricard
Ramsden	Rasul	Rebel	Remi	Reyes	Ricardo
Ramses	Rathal	Rebop	Remington	Reymond	Riccardo
Ramsey	Ratin	Rechavia	Remo	Reymundo	Ricci
Ramzey	Ratmir	Red	Remus	Reyn	Ricco
Ramzi	Rauf	Reda	Remy	Reynald	Rice
Ramzie	Raúl	Redd	Ren	Reynaldo	Rich
Ranald	Raulo	Redeemer	Renaldo	Reynard	Richard
Rance	Raum	Redell	Renard	Reynardo	Richardd
Rancher	Raunaeril	Redford	Renate	Reynold	Richardo
Rand	Rauvelore	Redley	Renato	Reza	Richart
Randal	Rave	Redman	Renatus	Rezalino	Richie
Randall	Raven	Redmond	Renau	Rezin	Richman
Randell	Ravi	Reece	Renaud	Rhaac'var	Richmond
Randi	Ravid	Reed	Rendor	Rhadamanthus	Rick
Randolph	Raviv	Reef	Rene	Rhalyf	Ricker
Randson	Ravon	Reegan	Renfield	Rhangyl	Rickey
Randy	Rawdon	Rees	Renfred	Rheged	Rickie
Ranell	Rawlins	Reese	Renfrew	Rhesus	Rickward
Ranen	Rawls	Reeve	Renjiro	Rhett	Ricky
Ranger	Rawson	Reeves	Renly	Rhinebeck	Rickyy
Rangle	Ray	Refive	Renne	Rhinelander	Rico
Rangsey	Rayan	Refugio	Rennie	Rhinffrew	Rida
Rani	Rayburn	Reg	Rennon	Rhioganedd	Ridder
Ranier	Rayce	Regan	Renny	Rhisiart	Rider
Ranit	Rayden	Reggie	Rennyn	Rhistel	Ridge
Ranjeet	Rayder	Regginald	Reno	Rhobert	Ridgeley
Ranjit	Raydon	Reginald	Renon	Rhodes	Ridgely
Rankin	Rayford	Regino	Renshaw	Rhodri	Ridgeway
Ranndy	Rayhan	Regis	Renton	Rhody	Ridha
Ranon	Raylan	Rego	Renwick	Rhory	Ridley
Ransford	Raylen	Rei	Renz	Rhoslyn	Ridwan
Ransley	Rayman	Reichan	Renzo	Rhothomir	Riel
Ransom	Raymon	Reid	Reo	Rhun	Rigby
Ranulf	Raymond	Reidar	Reon	Rhuvawn	Rigel
Ranulph	Raymund	Reign	Reptar	Rhyan	Rigg
Ranvir	Raymundo	Reijo	Requiem	Rhyawdd	Riggs
Raoul	Raynard	Reiki	Respen	Rhychdir	Rigny
Raphael	Rayne	Reilley	Reth	Rhyd	Rigoberto
Rapoto	Raynell	Reilly	Reuben	Rhydderch	Riki
Rashad	Rayner	Reinaldo	Reuel	Rhydian	Rikki

Riku	Robbert	Rodrigo	Romney	Rothilion	Ruddy
Rikuto	Robbie	Rodriguez	Romochka	Rothwell	Rudi
Riley	Robbin	Roe	Romolo	Rouchdy	Rudiger
Rilitar	Robby	Roel	Romulus	Rourke	Rudolf
Riluaneth	Robeert	Roep	Romy	Rousse	Rudolfo
Rimba	Roberrt	Rogan	Ron	Rousseau	Rudolph
Rimbo	Robert	Rogelio	Ronald	Roussel	Rudy
Rimon	Roberto	Rogene	Ronaldo	Rousset	Rudyard
Rin	Roberts	Roger	Ronan	Rousskin	Rue
Rinaldo	Robertson	Rogier	Rondel	Rouvin	Rueban
Ring	Robertt	Rogue	Rondell	Roux	Ruehar
Ringo	Robin	Rohaan	Ronel	Rover	Ruelle
Rinji	Robinson	Rohak	Ronell	Row	Rufaro
Rio	Robyn	Rohan	Ronen	Rowan	Ruff
Riobard	Roc	Rohit	Rong	Rowdon	Ruffe
Riodhr	Rocco	Rohmer	Roni	Rowdy	Ruffus
Rion	Roch	Roho	Ronin	Rowell	Rufin
Riordain	Roche	Roi	Ronit	Rowen	Rufino
Riordan	Rochester	Roibin	Ronn	Rowin	Rufio
Rip	Rocio	Rojelio	Ronnald	Rowland	Rufo
Ripley	Rock	Rojo	Ronnell	Rowley	Ruford
Rique	Rocke	Roka	Ronnie	Rowson	Rufus
Rishawn	Rockefeller	Rokuro	Ronny	Rowtag	Rugby
Rishi	Rocket	Rokurou	Ronson	Rowyn	Ruggero
Rishon	Rockley	Roland	Rook	Roxbert	Ruggiero
Risley	Rocklin	Rolando	Roone	Roxbury	Ruh
Risteard	Rocko	Roldan	Rooney	Roy	Ruhan
Risto	Rockwell	Rolf	Roosevelt	Royal	Rui
Riston	Rocky	Rolfe	Roper	Royan	Ruith
Ritchard	Rod	Rolim	Roque	Royce	Rujula
Ritchie	Rodas	Rollan	Roreto	Royd	Rule
Rito	Rodd	Rolland	Rorey	Royden	Rumba
Ritter	Rodderick	Rollie	Rorik	Royns	Rumenea
River	Roddney	Rollin	Rorke	Royston	Rumer
Rivera	Roddrick	Rollins	Rorric	Rozen	Rumford
Rives	Roddy	Rollo	Rorry	Ruadan	Rumo
Riyad	Rodel	Rolo	Rory	Ruadhagan	Rumor
Riyaz	Rodell	Rolphe	Rosario	Ruadhan	Rune
Rizwaan	Roden	Roma	Roscoe	Ruaidhri	Rungnir
Rizwan	Rodeo	Romain	Roselin	Ruanaidh	Runyon
Rizzo	Roderick	Roman	Roselyn	Ruarc	Rupert
Roald	Roderigo	Romano	Rosh	Ruardh	Rupin
Roan	Roderik	Romanus	Roshan	Ruark	Ruprecht
Roane	Roderrick	Romany	Roshaun	Rubben	Rurik
Roano	Rodger	Rome	Roslin	Ruben	Rush
Roark	Rodion	Romejin	Ross	Rubin	Rushe
Rob	Rodman	Romelo	Rossiter	Rubio	Rushford
Rob Roy	Rodney	Romeo	Rosston	Rubo	Rushil
Robb	Rodolfo	Romer	Rotem	Ruby	Rushkin
Robbe	Rodric	Romilly	Roth	Rudd	Rusk

Ruskin	Ryul	Saebeorht	Salih	Sanders	Satan
Ruslan	Ryuu	Saeed	Salil	Sanderson	Satchel
Russ	Ryuunosuke	Saelethil	Salim	Sandevv	Satin
Russel	Ryyan	Saer	Salinger	Sandhurst	Satordi
Russell	Ryzard	Saeran	Salisbury	Sanditon	Satoshi
Russo		Saevel	Salix	Sandler	Satria
Russom	**S**	Safari	Salman	Sandor	Satriya
Rust		Safford	Salmon	Sandrino	Saturday
Rusti		Saffron	Salmoneus	Sandro	Saturn
Ruston	Saa	Safi	Saloman	Sandros	Saturnin
Rusty	Saad	Sagan	Salomon	Sandy	Satya
Rusul	Saadiah	Sagar	Saloso	Sanford	Saul
Rutger	Saadya	Sage	Salton	Sanga	Sauts
Rutherford	Saahdia	Sagiv	Salus	Sani	Sauville
Rutland	Saam	Saguaro	Salvador	Sanjay	Sava
Rutledge	Saamir	Sahaj	Salvadore	Sanjaya	Saverio
Rutley	Saar	Sahak	Salvator	Sanjeet	Saviero
Ruvaen	Saarik	Sahale	Salvatore	Sanjiro	Saville
Ruven	Sabastian	Sahan	Salvatorio	Sanjiv	Savino
Ruvyn	Sabbath	Sahar	Salvino	Sanson	Savio
Ruzgar	Saber	Sahil	Salvio	Sansone	Savion
Ryaan	Sabik	Sahir	Sam	Santa	Savir
Ryan	Sabin	Sahrahsahe	Samad	Santana	Savoy
Ryatt	Sabino	Said	Samal	Santeri	Savva
Rychell	Sabir	Saidi	Saman	Santiago	Savyon
Rycroft	Sabiti	Saif	Samar	Santino	Sawyer
Ryden	Sable	Saiful	Samblar	Santo	Sawyers
Ryder	Sabo	Saifullah	Sambo	Santos	Sax
Rye	Sabra	Sail	Sami	Sanya	Saxe
Ryen	Sabre	Sailor	Samiir	Sanyu	Saxen
Ryfon	Sabri	Sainsbury	Samir	Sapir	Saxon
Ryker	Sabriel	Saint	Samm	Saqib	Saxton
Rylan	Saburo	Saith	Samman	Sarad	Sayer
Ryland	Saburou	Sajan	Sammie	Sardar	Sayers
Ryle	Sacha	Sajjad	Sammuel	Sargent	Sayid
Rylee	Sachar	Saka	Sammy	Sarki	Sayre
Ryleigh	Sachet	Sakari	Samo	Sarkis	Sayres
Rylen	Sacheverell	Sakarias	Samoel	Sarmad	Sayyid
Ryley	Sachi	Sakeri	Samoset	Saroyan	Scanlon
Rylie	Sachiel	Sakhr	Sampson	Sarpedon	Sceapleigh
Ryn	Sachin	Sakima	Samson	Sarto	Schaeffer
Ryne	Sachio	Saku	Samu	Sarva	Schatzi
Ryo	Sackville	Sal	Samuel	Sascha	Schmaiah
Ryoichi	Sadaf	Saladin	Samuell	Sasha	Schmuel
Ryon	Sadaka	Salah	Samuru	Sashenka	Schubert
Ryons	Saddam	Salamon	Samwell	Sason	Schultz
Ryosuke	Sadi	Salbatore	Sanborn	Sassaba	Schuyler
Ryota	Sadik	Saleem	Sancho	Sassacus	Schylar
Ryoto	Sadiki	Saleh	Sandberg	Sasson	Schyler
Ryu	Sadler	Salem	Sander	Sasuke	Science
	Sadwm				

Scipio	Sef	Seosaph	Shaad	Shani	Shelly
Scirocco	Seferino	September	Shaan	Shanley	Shelomo
Sclymgeour	Seff	Septimus	Shabaan	Shann	Shelton
Scoop	Sefton	Sequence	Shabat	Shannan	Shem
Scooter	Segenam	Sequester	Shachar	Shannen	Shemar
Scopas	Seger	Sequin	Shad	Shannon	Shemus
Scorpio	Seghen	Sequoia	Shadan	Shapur	Shenandoah
Scot	Segundo	Sequoyah	Shadd	Shaqir	Sheng
Scott	Seibert	Serafim	Shade	Shaquille	Shep
Scottie	Seifer	Serafin	Shadi	Shareef	Shepherd
Scotty	Seignour	Seraiah	Shadow	Shariah	Shepley
Scout	Seiji	Seraphim	Shadrach	Sharian	Sher
Scribner	Seiko	Seren	Shae	Sharif	Sheraga
Scully	Sein	Sereno	Shael	Shashenka	Sherborn
Seabert	Seireadan	Serge	Shafaqat	Shashi	Sheridan
Seabroc	Seith	Sergeant	Shafiq	Shasta	Sherif
Seabrook	Seiveril	Sergei	Shafir	Shauden	Sherill
Seaburt	Sekou	Sergio	Shahab	Shaughn	Sherlock
Seabury	Sel	Sergios	Shahaka	Shaul	Sherman
Seafra	Sela	Sergius	Shaham	Shaun	Sheron
Seafraid	Selanlar	Sergiusz	Shahan	Shaundre	Sherrerd
Seaghda	Selas	Serguei	Shahar	Shaundyl	Sherwin
Seaghdha	Selatan	Seriozha	Shahin	Shaunn	Sherwood
Seagull	Selby	Seriozhenka	Shahnaz	Shaviv	Shet
Seal	Seldon	Servan	Shahryar	Shavon	Sheva
Sealey	Selgauth	Servas	Shahzad	Shavtiel	Shey
Seaman	Selig	Set	Shai	Shaw	Shia
Seamore	Selik	Seth	Shain	Shawano	Shichiro
Seamus	Selkirk	Setia	Shaine	Shawe	Shichirou
Sean	Sellers	Seton	Shaka	Shawn	Shields
Seanan	Selvyn	Seumas	Shaked	Shawnee	Shihab
Searlas	Selwyn	Sevan	Shakespeare	Shawnel	Shikamaru
Searle	Selyf	Sevastian	Shakil	Shawnn	Shilah
Searlus	Selyv	Seven	Shakir	Shay	Shilo
Seath	Sem	Severin	Shaktar	Shaya	Shiloah
Seaton	Semaj	Severino	Shale	Shayan	Shiloh
Seb	Seminole	Severn	Shalev	Shayde	Shimmel
Sebasten	Semyon	Severne	Shalom	Shaye	Shimon
Sebastiaan	Sender	Severo	Shaman	Shaylon	Shimshon
Sebastian	Seneca	Severus	Shamar	Shayne	Shin
Sebastiano	Senegal	Sevilen	Shamil	Shea	Shing
Scbasticn	Sencn	Sevrin	Shamir	Sheadon	Shinjiro
Sebert	Senet	Seward	Shamus	Sheary	Shino
Secondo	Senior	Sewati	Shan	Shecayah	Shinobu
Sedgeley	Sennet	Sewell	Shanahan	Sheehan	Shinsaku
Sedgely	Sennett	Seweryn	Shandar	Sheffield	Shinta
Sedgley	Senon	Sexton	Shandon	Shel	Shipley
Sedgwick	Senya	Sextus	Shandy	Shelby	Shipton
Seeger	Seoras	Seyah	Shane	Sheldon	Shiriki
Seeley	Seosamh	Seymour	Shango	Shelley	Shiro

Shiron	Siddel	Simba	Skate	Soma	Spiridon
Shirou	Siddhartha	Simcha	Skeet	Somer	Spiro
Shiva	Sidharth	Simen	Skelly	Somerby	Sprague
Shiye	Sidney	Simeon	Skelton	Somerley	Sprig
Shizhe'e	Sidonio	Simimar	Skene	Somers	Springer
Shlomo	Sidonus	Simm	Skerry	Somerset	Spruce
Shmaryahu	Siegfried	Simmon	Skinner	Somerton	Spud
Shmuel	Siencyn	Simmons	Skip	Somerville	Spyridon
Shmuley	Sierra	Simon	Skipper	Son	Squall
Sho	Sigbjorn	Simpson	Skule	Songaa	Squire
Shoda	Sigfried	Sims	Sky	Sonnagh	Sroel
Shogo	Sigifrid	Simson	Skye	Sonnet	Stacey
Shohei	Sigifrith	Sina	Skyelar	Sonnie	Stacy
Sholto	Sigismondo	Sinaht	Skylar	Sonny	Staffan
Shomecossee	Sigmond	Sinai	Skyler	Sontar	Stafford
Shomer	Sigmund	Sinan	Skylor	Sophocles	Stamatios
Shoneah	Signe	Sinasta	Slade	Sora	Stamitos
Shoney	Sigourney	Sinbad	Slate	Sorel	Stamos
Shonka	Sigurd	Sincere	Slater	Soren	Stan
Shonn	Sigvard	Sinclair	Slavik	Sorley	Stanbury
Shooter	Sigwald	Sinclaire	Slavin	Sorrel	Stancio
Shoshone	Sigwalt	Sindre	Slavomir	Sorrell	Stancliff
Shou	Siimon	Sindri	Slim	Sorren	Standish
Shouta	Siirist	Sinjin	Sloan	Sosthenes	Stanfield
Shoval	Sik'is	Sinjon	Sloane	Soterios	Stanford
Shoya	Sike	Sinnoch	Slone	Sothern	Stanislas
Shraga	Sikyahonaw	Sinon	Sly	Sotirios	Stanislaus
Shu	Sikyatavo	Siomon	Smedley	Sotiris	Stanislav
Shuang	Sil	Sion	Smit	Soto	Stanislaw
Shubha	Silas	Sionn	Smith	Sotsona	Stanislov
Shudra	Silence	Sior	Smokey	Souta	Stanko
Shui	Silko	Siraj	Smoky	Southern	Stanley
Shukri	Sill	Sirius	Smyth	Southwell	Stanmore
Shulamith	Silos	Siro	Snowden	Soutine	Stannes
Shun	Silvain	Sisqó	Snowy	Sovann	Stannis
Shunpei	Silvano	Sisyphus	Snyder	Sowi'ngwa	Stanton
Shura	Silvanus	Sitanka	Sobhi	Spalding	Stanway
Shurik	Silver	Siv	Socorro	Spark	Stanwick
Shurochka	Silverio	Sivan	Socrates	Sparrow	Stanwood
Shuya	Silverman	Sivney	Sofer	Spartacus	Star
Shyam	Silverton	Siwili	Sofronio	Spear	Starbuck
Shyrrik	Silvester	Sixsipita	Sofus	Speck	Stark
Siâm	Silvestre	Sixte	Sohan	Speed	Starlin
Siard	Silvijn	Sixten	Soho	Speedy	Starling
Siarl	Silvino	Sixtus	Sojourner	Spence	Starr
Siawn	Silvio	Siyamak	Sol	Spencer	Stash
Sibley	Silvius	Siyavash	Solaris	Spenser	Stav
Sicheii	Silvyr	Skah	Soleh	Spicer	Stavros
Sicily	Sim	Skalanis	Solomon	Spider	Stavya
Sid	Simao	Skanawati	Solon	Spike	Steadman

Steafan	Stew	Suguru	Sweden	Tabor	Taj
Stedman	Stewart	Sugyn	Sweeney	Tacey	Taji
Steed	Sthir	Suhayl	Swinburne	Tacitus	Tajo
Steef	Stian	Suhul	Swindel	Tacy	Takahiro
Steel	Stig	Suibhne	Swinford	Tad	Takashi
Steele	Stijn	Suileabhan	Swinton	Tadao	Takashia
Steeve	Stiles	Sujay	Swithbert	Tadd	Takato
Steeven	Stille	Sulaiman	Swithin	Taddeo	Takehiko
Stefan	Stillman	Sulayman	Swithun	Tadelesh	Takeo
Stefano	Stirling	Sulien	Sy	Taden	Takeshi
Stefanos	Stockard	Sullivan	Syaoran	Tadeo	Takis
Steffan	Stockley	Sully	Syd	Tadhg	Takoda
Steffano	Stockton	Sultan	Sydnee	Tadi	Takuma
Steffen	Stockwell	Sulyen	Sydney	Tadleigh	Takumi
Steffon	Stoddard	Suman	Syed	Taegen	Takuya
Stefford	Stoker	Sumarville	Sylas	Taenaran	Tal
Stefon	Stone	Sumeet	Syler	Taeral	Talan
Stein	Stoney	Summer	Sylvain	Taerntym	Talasi
Steinar	Storm	Sumner	Sylvan	Tafari	Talbet
Stellan	Stormy	Sun	Sylvar	Taffy	Talbot
Stellen	Story	Sundamar	Sylvester	Taft	Talcott
Steltella	Stover	Sunday	Symeon	Tag	Taleb
Sten	Stowe	Sundown	Symkalr	Tage	Talehot
Stennis	Stoyan	Sunesh	Symon	Taggart	Taleisin
Step	Strahan	Sunil	Synclair	Tahan	Talen
Steph	Stratford	Sunny	Syon	Tahbert	Talfryn
Stephan	Straus	Suoh	Syrus	Tahigwa	Talib
Stephano	Street	Surya	Syshe	Tahir	Taliesin
Stephanos	Strickland	Susila	Sythaeryn	Tahkeome	Tallis
Stephanus	Striker	Susumu	Syvwkh	Tahmel	Tallon
Stephen	Strom	Sutcliff	Szczepan	Tahmid	Tallys
Stephenson	Strong	Sutherland		Tahmores	Talmadge
Stephon	Struan	Sutter	**T**	Tahoe	Talmai
Stepka	Struthers	Sutton		Tahoma	Talman
Stepney	Stryker	Suvan	Taanyth	Tahsin	Talmon
Sterlin	Stu	Suzu	Taariq	Tahu	Talon
Sterling	Stuart	Svatomir	Taaveti	Tai	Talos
Sterne	Studs	Svatoslav	Taavetti	Tai Yang	Talus
Stesha	Styles	Svein	Taavi	Taichi	Talyessin
Stetson	Suave	Sven	Taavon	Taicligh	Tam
Stevan	Subhan	Svend	Tab	Taiden	Tamaki
Steve	Sucki	Svens	Taban	Taifa	Taman
Steveland	Sudbury	Sverre	Tabananica	Taijo	Tamar
Steven	Sudryl	Swahili	Tabari	Taiki	Tamarack
Stevenn	Suede	Swain	Tabasco	Taillefer	Tamarisk
Stevens	Suelita	Swaine	Tabassum	Taima	Tamary
Stevenson	Suffield	Swaley	Tabbart	Taiomah	Tamas
Steverino	Suffolk	Swann	Taber	Taisce	Tambe
Stevie	Sufjan	Swannee	Tabib	Tait	Tamerlaine
Stevyn	Sugden	Swanton	Tabner	Taite	Tamerlane

55

Tameron	Taran	Taurino	Ted	Teo	Thacker
Tamesis	Taranath	Tauro	Tedd	Teodor	Thackeray
Tamir	Tarasios	Taurus	Teddington	Teodoro	Thad
Tamjid	Tarathiel	Tausiq	Teddy	Teodors	Thaddeus
Tamlane	Taredd	Tavaris	Tedmund	Teofile	Thaddius
Tammany	Taregan	Tavarius	Tedric	Teom	Thadeus
Tamnaeuth	Tarek	Tavarris	Tedrick	Teos	Thady
Tamryn	Taren	Tave	Tedros	Teppo	Thai
Tamson	Tareq	Taveon	Teel	Terach	Thais
Tan	Tarhe	Taverner	Teenie	Terciero	Thalanil
Tanav	Tarian	Tavey	Teetonka	Teregud	THALES
Tanay	Tarin	Tavi	Tefo	Terence	Thallan
Tanchum	Tariq	Tavian	Tehlmar	Terika	Thaman
Tancred	Tarleton	Tavin	Teige	Teris	Thanatos
Tancredo	Tarlo	Tavio	Teiji	Tern	Thandiwe
Tandie	Tarmo	Tavion	Teilo	Terran	Thane
Tandy	Tarmon	Tavis	Teirist	Terrance	Thangbrand
Tane	Taro	Tavish	Teithi	Terre	Thanh
Taneli	Taron	Tavon	Tejano	Terrel	Thanos
Taner	Tarot	Tavonn	Telamon	Terrell	Tharin
Tangakwunu	Tarou	Tavor	Telegonus	Terrelle	Thatcher
Tangier	Tarquin	Tavorian	Telek	Terrence	Thaumas
Tango	Tarran	Taworri	Telemachus	Terrian	Thaw
Tanguy	Tarrant	Tay	Telephus	Terrin	Thaxter
Taniel	Tarrence	Tayanita	Telfer	Terris	Thayer
Tanishia	Tarrik	Tayden	Telfor	Terriss	Thel
Tanithil	Tarron	Taye	Telford	Terron	Thelonious
Tanix	Taru	Tayeb	Telfour	Terry	Thelonius
Tanjiro	Tarun	Taylan	Teller	Terryal	Thelred
Tannar	Tarver	Tayler	Tellus	Tertius	Themba
Tanner	Taryn	Taylon	Telly	Teshi	Theo
Tannin	Tarzan	Taylor	Telmo	Tetley	Theobald
Tannivh	Tas	Tayson	Telutci	Teton	Theoclymenus
Tannon	Tasar	Tayte	Teman	Tetsuya	Theodon
Tanny	Tascalusa	Tayten	Temani	Teun	Theodore
Tannyll	Tasha	Tayton	Tempest	Teuthras	Theodoric
Tantalus	Tassarion	Tayyib	Temple	Teva	Theodosios
Tanton	Tasso	Taz	Templeton	Tevin	Theodrekr
Tanwyn	Tassos	Tchondee	Tempo	Tevis	Theodric
Tanya	Tasunke	Teagan	Temujin	Tevon	Theodrik
Tanyl	Tate	Teaghue	Tenauri	Tevya	Theon
Tao	Tatenda	Teague	Tene	Tew	Theophile
Taos	Tathaln	Teal	Teneil	Tewdwr	Theophilos
Tapa	Tatsuhiro	Teale	Tenen	Tex	Theophilus
Tapani	Tatsuya	Teangi	Tennant	Texas	Theoris
Tapio	Tattuye	Tearlach	Tennessee	Teyemthohisa	Therius
Tappen	Tatum	Tearley	Tennis	Teyo	Theron
Tarachand	Tau	Tearly	Tennyson	Tezcacoatl	Therron
Tarafah	Tauankia	Teauge	Tenoch	Thabit	Thersites
Tarak	Taurean	Tecumseh	Tenskwatawa	Thackary	Theseus

Thessaly	Thurman	Timo	Tohkieto	Toraidio	Toussaint
Thiago	Thurstan	Timocrates	Tohopka	Toran	Toussnint
Thian	Thurston	Timofey	Tohy	Torben	Tove
Thibaud	Thutmose	Timoleon	Toivo	Tordynnar	Tovi
Thibault	Thuyet	Timon	Tokala	Torean	Toviel
Thieny	Thwaite	Timoteo	Tokori	Toren	Tower
Thierry	Thyestes	Timotheos	Tokyo	Torence	Townsend
Thiery	Tiago	Timotheus	Tolan	Torey	Toxeus
Thijmen	Tianna	Timothhy	Toland	Torgeir	Trace
Thijs	Tiarchnach	Timothy	Tolek	Torger	Tracen
Thimba	Tiarshus	Timothyy	Tolenka	Torgny	Tracey
Thjalfi	Tiassale	Timun	Toli	Torhte	Track
Thom	Tibault	Timur	Toller	Toril	Tracy
Thoma	Tibbot	Tino	Tolliver	Torin	Trader
Thomas	Tiberio	Tiomoid	Toltecatl	Torio	Trae
Thomass	Tiberius	Tip	Tolthe	Torion	Traeliorn
Thommas	Tibone	Tipu	Tolya	Tormaigh	Trahaym
Thompson	Tibor	Tiran	Tom	Tormey	Trahern
Thono	Tiburon	Tiras	Tomai	Torn	Trai
Thor	Tide	Titan	Tomaisin	Toro	Traigh
Thorald	Tiebout	Tithonus	Tomas	Torolf	Trail
Thorbert	Tiege	Tito	Tomasso	Toross	Tramaine
Thorbiartl	Tier	Titos	Tomasz	Torquil	Trapper
Thorburn	Tiergan	Titus	Tomek	Torr	Traugott
Thoreau	Tiernan	Tityus	Tomeo	Torran	Trautwein
Thoren	Tiernay	Tivadar	Tomer	Torrance	Travaran
Thorgils	Tierney	Tivon	Tomi	Torrans	Traveler
Thorin	Tige	Tkalis	Tomislaw	Torre	Traveon
Thorley	Tiger	Tlacelel	Tomlin	Torrell	Travers
Thormond	Tigernach	Tlannatar	Tomm	Torrence	Travion
Thorndike	Tighe	Toan	Tommaso	Torrey	Travis
Thorndyke	Tihalt	Tobal	Tommen	Torrian	Traviss
Thorne	Tihkoosue	Tobby	Tommy	Torrie	Travon
Thornley	Tikhon	Tobey	Tomos	Torrin	Travonn
Thornlie	Tilak	Tobiah	Tomoya	Torry	Tray
Thornton	Tilden	Tobias	Tompkins	Torsten	Traylor
Thornycroft	Tilford	Tobin	Toms	Toru	Trayton
Thorpe	Till	Toby	Ton	Torvald	Tre
Thorstein	Tillman	Tobyn	Toney	Tory	Trea
Thorsten	Tillmann	Tocho	Toni	Toryn	Treabhar
Thorvid	Tiltilla	Tochtli	Tonio	Toseland	Treacy
Thu	Tilton	Tod	Tonny	Toshawah	Treasach
Thule	Tim	Todd	Tony	Toshihiro	Treasigh
Thunder	Timaeus	Toddy	Tooantuh	Toshio	Treat
Thuong	Timber	Todhunter	Topaz	Toshiro	Tremain
Thurber	Timeo	Todor	Topher	Tostig	Tremaine
Thurdan	Timeus	Toft	Topi	Tosya	Tremayne
Thurgood	Timm	Togo	Topias	Totole	Tremen
Thurl	Timmothy	Togquos	Topper	Toulouse	Tremont
Thurlow	Timmy	Tohias	Tor	Toure	Trenner

57

Trent	Trout	Tupi	Tyquann	Udeh	Uranus
Trenten	Trowbridge	Tupper	Tyr	Udell	Urbain
Trenton	Trowbrydge	Turannos	Tyran	Udi	Urban
Treowbrycg	Troy	Turbo	Tyreak	Udo	Urbano
Treoweman	Troyes	Turi	Tyree	Udolf	Urddusk
Trevan	Tru	Turk	Tyreece	Uehudah	Urho
Trevelian	Trudord	Turner	Tyreek	Uevareth	Uri
Trevelyan	Truesdale	Turtle	Tyrek	Ugo	Uriah
Treven	Truls	Tusya	Tyrel	Ugra	Urian
Trever	Truman	Tut	Tyrell	Ugur	Urie
Treves	Trumble	Tutyahu	Tyrelle	Uilleam	Uriel
Trevet	Trumen	Tuve	Tyren	Uilliam	Urien
Trevian	Trumhall	Tuvia	Tyrese	Uisdean	Uriens
Trevin	Trung	Tuvya	Tyrion	Uja	Urijah
Trevion	Truong	Twain	Tyrique	Ukiah	Urso
Trevis	Trust	Twiford	Tyrone	Ulan	Usain
Trevls	Truth	Twila	Tyronn	Uldreiyn	Usama
Trevon	Trygg	Twilight	Tyronne	Ulema	Usamah
Trevonn	Trygve	Twitchel	Tyrrel	Ulf	Usbeorn
Trevor	Trymian	Twm	Tyrrell	Ulfred	Usher
Trevvor	Trymman	Twrgadarn	Tyrus	Uli	Ushi
Trevyn	Trynt	Twyford	Tyshawn	Ulick	Usman
Trey	Trystan	Ty	Tyson	Ulises	Uso
Treyton	Tsar	Tybalt	Tythan	Ull	Ustin
Treyvon	Tsidhqiyah	Tyce	Tyvan	Ulmer	Usunaar
Tri	Tsiyone	Tycho	Tywin	Ulric	Utah
Triage	Tsubasa	Tychon	Tywysog	Ulrich	Utara
Triandal	Tsungani	Tydeus	Tzadok	Ultan	Utcha
Trig	Tsuyoshi	Tye	Tzefaniah	Ulysses	Uther
Trigg	Tsvetan	Tyee	Tzefanyah	Umar	Uthman
Trilby	Tu	Tyeis	Tzefanyahu	Umber	Uthorim
Tringad	Tuan	Tyeson	Tzion	Umberto	Uttam
Trip	Tuari	Tyfiell	Tziyon	Umed	Uz
Tripada	Tucker	Tygo	Tzuriel	Umi	Uzi
Tripp	Tucson	Tyipa	Tzvi	Umut	Uziah
Triptolemus	Tudor	Tylar		Unai	Uziel
Tristam	Tuesday	Tyler	**U**	Uncas	Uzumati
Tristan	Tufayl	Tylissus		Ungus	Uzziah
Tristen	Tuketu	Tylor	Uaid	Uni	Uzziel
Tristian	Tulio	Tym	Uaine	Unika	
Tristin	Tullio	Tyme	Ualair	Unique	**V**
Triston	Tullis	Tymek	Ualtar	Unwin	
Tristram	Tullius	Tymon	Uba	Uorsin	Vaalyun
Tristyn	Tully	Tynan	Ubadah	Upchurch	Vachel
Triton	Tumaini	Tyndareus	Ubaydullah	Updike	Vaclav
Troian	Tumenah	Tyne	Uberto	Upendo	Václav
Troilus	Tumo	Typhoeus	Uchdryd	Upshaw	Vaddon
Trophonius	Tune	Typhon	Uchenna	Upton	Vadim
Trory	Tuomo	Typhoon	Uday	Upwood	Vadin
Trot	Tupac	Tyquan	Udayan	Ura	Vaeril

Vahe	Vardinon	Veltry	Viator	Vinny	Vontell
Vahn	Vardon	Velvel	Vic	Vinson	Voron
Vail	Vareck	Vemados	Vice	Vinton	Vortimer
Vaiveahtoish	Varek	Venali	Vicente	Vipponah	Voshell
Vajra	Varen	Venamin	Vick	Viral	Voss
Val	Varian	Venedict	Vicky	Virendra	Vox
Valdemar	Varick	Venedictos	Vicq	Vireo	Vrai
Vale	Varik	Venezio	Victor	Virgil	Vulcan
Valen	Varius	Veniamin	Victoriano	Virgilio	Vulmaro
Valente	Varro	Venjamin	Victorien	Virginius	Vyacheslav
Valentin	Vartan	Venn	Victorin	Virgo	Vychan
Valentine	Varten	Venturi	Victorino	Viridian	
Valentino	Varun	Venturo	Victorio	Virote	

W

Valera	Varuna	Venu	Victoro	Vischer	
Valerian	Vas	Venya	Vicus	Viserys	Waapalaa
Valerii	Vasant	Veradis	Vidal	Vishnu	Wabanang
Valerik	Vaschel	Verddun	Vidar	Vital	Wade
Valerio	Vasco	Verdell	Videl	Vitale	Wadee
Valerius	Vasha	Verdi	Vidor	Vitalis	Wadham
Valeriy	Vashon	Vere	Viet	Vitaliy	Wadley
Valery	Vasileios	Vered	Viggo	Vitaly	Wadsworth
Valhalla	Vasili	Verel	Vigo	Vitenka	Wadu
Vali	Vasilii	Vergil	Vihaan	Vito	Wael
Valiant	Vasilios	Verlee	Viho	Vittorio	Waerheall
Valin	Vasilis	Verlyn	Vijay	Viturin	Wafa
Valko	Vasiliy	Vermont	Vikram	Vitus	Wafai
Vallen	Vasily	Vern	Viktor	Vivaldo	Wafi
Vallis	Vasin	Vernados	Vila	Vivek	Waggoner
Vallois	Vasos	Vernay	Vilhelm	Vivian	Wagner
Valmiki	Vassar	Verne	Viliam	Viviano	Wahanassatta
Valo	Vassi	Vernell	Viliulfo	Vivien	Wahchinksapa
Valor	Vassily	Verner	Viljo	Vlad	Wahchintonka
Valter	Vasska	Verneri	Villard	Vladik	Waheed
Valthjof	Vasya	Verney	Villiers	Vladilen	Wahib
Valtteri	Vasyltso	Vernon	Vilmos	Vladimir	Wahid
Vaman	Vasyklo	Vero	Vin	Vladislav	Wahkan
Van	Vasyl	Verrall	Vinay	Vladmir	Wahmenitu
Vance	Vatsa	Verrell	Vince	Vladmiri	Wain
Vandal	Vaughan	Verrier	Vincens	Vladya	Wainwright
Vander	Vaughn	Verrill	Vincent	Vohkinne	Waite
Vandyke	Vayle	Veryl	Vincente	Voistitoevitz	Wajid
Vane	Vayu	Vesper	Vincenzio	Volante	Wakapa
Vanechka	Ved	Vesperr	Vincenzo	Volker	Wakaun
Vanhi	Veda	Vesryn	Vinci	Volney	Wake
Vanir	Veer	Vesstan	Vine	Volodar	Wakechai
Vanya	Vega	Vester	Vineet	Volody	Wakefield
Vanyusha	Vegar	Vesuvio	Ving	Volsung	Wakeley
Varan	Vegard	Veto	Vinicio	Von	Wakely
Vardan	Veit	Vevay	Vinn	Vonn	Wakeman
Varden	Velethuil	Vian	Vinnie	Vonte	Wakichonze

Wakinyela	Waqar	Weatherby	Westin	Wilfred	Winthrop
Wakiza	Waquini	Weaver	Westley	Wilfredo	Winton
Walbridge	Warburton	Weayaya	Weston	Wilhelm	Winwodem
Walbrydge	Ward	Webb	Wetherby	Wilkes	Winwood
Walby	Wardell	Webber	Wetherell	Wilkie	Wirecaster
Walcott	Warden	Webley	Wetherly	Wilkins	Wirt
Wald	Wardley	Webster	Wevers	Wilkinson	Wisconsin
Waldemar	Ware	Wedgwood	Weyland	Will	Wistar
Walden	Warfield	Wednesday	Weylin	Willa	Wistari
Waldifrid	Warford	Wegland	Weylyn	Willard	Wit
Waldmunt	Warick	Wei	Wharton	Willem	Witt
Waldo	Warley	Weissman	Wheatley	Willesone	Witte
Waldon	Warner	Welborn	Wheaton	Willet	Wizard
Waldorf	Warrane	Welborne	Wheeler	Willfred	Wm
Waldron	Warren	Welby	Wheelwright	Willfredo	Wimm
Waldwick	Warrick	Weldon	Whistler	William	Wmffre
Walerian	Warton	Welford	Whit	Williams	Woape
Waleron	Wartun	Wellington	Whitbeck	Willie	Wohehiv
Wales	Warwick	Wells	Whitby	Willis	Woksapiwi
Walford	Wasabe	Welsh	Whitcomb	Willmar	Wolcott
Walfred	Wasaki	Welton	White	Willoughby	Wole
Walfrid	Waseem	Wematin	Whitehead	Willow	Wolf
Walid	Washakie	Wemilat	Whitelaw	Wills	Wolfe
Waljan	Washburn	Wen	Whitey	Willson	Wolfert
Walker	Washburne	Wenceslas	Whitfield	Willy	Wolfgang
Wallace	Washi	Wenceslaus	Whitford	Wilmer	Wolfric
Waller	Washington	Wenczeslaw	Whitlam	Wilmet	Wolverine
Wallis	Wasi	Wendale	Whitlaw	Wilmod	Wood
Wally	Wasim	Wendall	Whitley	Wilson	Woodrow
Walmond	Wassim	Wendel	Whitlock	Wilton	Woods
Walsh	Wataru	Wendelin	Whitman	Wim	Woodson
Walt	Watchemonne	Wendell	Whitmore	WiMor	Woodstock
Walter	Watelford	Wendlesora	Whitney	Win	Woodward
Waltham	Waterford	Wenopa	Whittaker	Wincent	Woody
Walton	Watkins	Wensley	Whoopi	Winchell	Woolworth
Walvia	Watson	Wentworth	Wiatt	Windell	Worcester
Walworth	Watt	Werhar	Wicasa	Windsor	Worth
Walwyn	Watts	Werner	Wickham	Winetorp	Wortham
Wamblee	Waunakee	Werther	Wickley	Winfield	Worthy
Wambleesha	Waverley	Wes	Wicus	Winfred	Worton
Wamukota	Waverly	Weshcubb	Wielladun	Wing	Wouter
Wanageeska	Wawinges	Weslan	Wienczyslaw	Wingate	Wowashi
Wanahton	Wayde	Wesley	Wigman	Winka	Woyzeck
Wanamaker	Waylan	Wesly	Wikvaya	Winn	Wozhupiwi
Wanbli	Wayland	Wessley	Wilbert	Winslow	Wray
Wanikiy	Waylon	West	Wilbur	Winsor	Wrecker
Wanyecha	Wayne	Westbrook	Wild	Winsted	Wren
Wapaheo	Waynne	Westby	Wilder	Winston	Wright
Wapi	Wealaworth	Westcott	Wiley	Wintanweorth	Wrisley
Wapiti	Weard	Westerly	Wilford	Winter	Wriston

Wuyi	Xanto	Yael	Yarran	Yeshaya	Yosemite
Wyandanch	Xarles	Yagil	Yarrow	Yeshayahu	Yoshi
Wyatt	Xavi	Yagmur	Yas	Yestin	Yoshiki
Wybert	Xaviar	Yago	Yasahiro	Yevgeni	Yoshirou
Wyck	Xavier	Yahir	Yaseen	Yevgeny	Yoshiteru
Wyckoff	Xavior	Yaholo	Yasen	Yhendorn	Yotam
Wyclef	Xen	Yahto	Yaser	Yiftach	Young
Wycliff	Xeno	Yahya	Yash	Yigal	Yousef
Wycombe	Xenon	Yair	Yasha	Yigil	Yovanny
Wyeth	Xenophon	Yakar	Yasiel	Yigol	Yoyko
Wylan	Xenos	Yakim	Yasir	Yildiz	Yrjö
Wylchyr	Xerxes	Yakir	Yasser	Yimeyam	Ysberin
Wylei	Xever	Yakov	Yasu	Yisachar	Ysgawyn
Wyler	Xhaiden	Yakub	Yasunari	Yishachar	Ysrael
Wylie	Xhalh	Yalathanil	Yasuo	Yishai	Yu
Wyman	Xhalth	Yale	Yates	Yiska	Yucatan
Wymer	Xharlion	Yama	Yatin	Yisrael	Yuda
Wyn	Xi-wang	Yamal	Yavin	Yisreal	Yudai
Wyndham	Xiao Chen	Yamir	Yavor	Yissachar	Yudel
Wynn	Xidorn	Yamparti	Yaxha	Yitro	Yue
Wynne	Ximen	Yan	Yazid	Yitzchak	Yue Yan
Wynono	Ximenes	Yanai	Ye	Yitzhak	Yuichi
Wynonom	Ximon	Yancey	Yeardleigh	Ylyndar	Yuki
Wynston	Ximun	Yancy	Yeardley	Ymir	Yukia
Wynter	Xing	Yandel	Yeats	Yngve	Yukio
Wynton	Xio	Yanis	Yechezkel	Yngwie	Yukon
Wyome	Xiomar	Yanisin	Yechiel	Ynyr	Yul
Wyoming	Xipil	Yaniv	Yedidiah	Yoad	Yule
Wyrran	Xiuhcoatl	Yank	Yedidyah	Yoav	Yuma
Wystan	Xola	Yankee	Yeeshai	Yochai	Yura
Wythe	Xorn	Yankel	Yefrem	Yochanan	Yurem
	Xuan	Yann	Yehoash	Yoda	Yuri
X	Xuthus	Yanni	Yehonadov	Yoel	Yurii
	Xylander	Yannick	Yehonatan	Yoelvis	Yurik
	Xylon	Yannis	Yehor	Yogi	Yuriy
Xabat	Xzavier	Yantse	Yehoshua	Yohance	Yurochka
Xadrian		Yaotl	Yehuda	Yoite	Yusef
Xaiver	**Y**	Yaotle	Yehudah	Yolotli	Yusei
Xakery		Yaphet	Yehudi	Yomtov	Yussuf
Xalbador		Yaqub	Yenge	Yon	Yusuf
Xalph	Yaacov	Yardan	Yeoman	Yonah	Yuta
Xalvador	Yaakov	Yardane	Yerachmiel	Yonas	Yuuki
Xan	Yaal	Yarden	Yered	Yonatan	Yuuta
Xanadu	Yaar	Yardley	Yeriel	Yoomee	Yuval
Xander	Yacoub	Yarema	Yerik	Yoram	Yuvraj
Xandy	Yada	Yaremka	Yermiyahu	Yorath	Yuya
Xannon	Yadid	Yarin	Yerodin	Yorick	Yves
Xanotter	Yadiel	Yaro	Yerucham	York	Yvet
Xanthos	Yadin	Yaron	Yeschant	Yosef	Yvian
Xanthus	Yadon	Yaroslav	Yesenin	Yosefu	Yvon
Xanti	Yaeger				

Z

Zaaire
Zabbas
Zabe
Zabi
Zabulon
Zac
Zacarias
Zacary
Zaccary
Zacchaeus
Zacchary
Zaccheo
Zaccheus
Zaccur
Zach
Zachaios
Zachalie
Zacharee
Zachariah
Zacharias
Zacharry
Zachary
Zachely
Zachery
Zaci
Zack
Zackary
Zackery
Zad
Zade
Zaden
Zadock
Zadok
Zadornin
Zafar
Zahar
Zahari
Zahavi
Zahi
Zahir
Zahn
Zahur
Zaid
Zaide
Zaiden
Zaidin
Zailey

Zaim
Zain
Zair
Zaire
Zajac
Zak
Zakai
Zakari
Zakaria
Zakary
Zakhar
Zaki
Zakiya
Zakk
Zakkary
Zako
Zale
Zalmai
Zalman
Zaltarish
Zamiel
Zamir
Zan
Zander
Zandophen
Zandro
Zandy
Zane
Zani
Zaor
Zaos
Zarad
Zareb
Zared
Zareh
Zarek
Zarney
Zarren
Zasha
Zavad
Zavid
Zavier
Zayd
Zayden
Zayit
Zayn
Zayne
Zazu
Zbigniew
Zeal

Zealand
Zeb
Zebadiah
Zebedee
Zebedeo
Zebediah
Zebidiah
Zebulan
Zebulon
Zebulun
Zecharia
Zechariah
Zed
Zedekiah
Zedhryx
Zeeman
Zeév
Zeger
Zeke
Zeki
Zelig
Zelimir
Zeljko
Zell
Zelmo
Zelotes
Zelozelos
Zelphar
Zen
Zenas
Zene
Zenebe
Zenith
Zenjiro
Zeno
Zenobio
Zenobios
Zenon
Zenos
Zenshiro
Zentaro
Zentavious
Zeo
Zephan
Zephaniah
Zephariah
Zephyr
Zephyrin
Zeppelin
Zerach

Zerah
Zero
Zeroun
Zerrick
Zerro
Zeru
Zeshawn
Zesiro
Zeta
Zetes
Zethus
Zeus
Zev
Zevadiah
Zevi
Zevon
Zevulun
Zhenechka
Zhenya
Zhi
Zhivago
Zhorah
Zhoron
Zhubin
Zia
Ziff
Ziggy
Zigor
Ziion
Zikomo
Zilya
Zimra
Zimran
Zimri
Zinc
Zindel
Zinedine
Zion
Zionn
Zipkiyah
Zitkaduta
Zitomir
Ziv
Ziven
Zivon
Ziya
Zo
Zoan
Zody
Zohar

Zoilo
Zola
Zoltan
Zoltar
Zolten
Zoltin
Zooey
Zophar
Zorba
Zorea
Zorion
Zory
Zotico
Zu
Zuberi
Zubin
Zuhayr
Zulimar
Zulu
Zuma
Zuni
Zuri
Zuriel
Zvi
Zwi
Zyler
Zytaveon

Girls Names

A

Aada
Aadi
Aafje
Aaid
Aalia
Aaliyah
Aallotar
Aaltje
Aamanda
Aamani
Aamber
Aamiya
Aana
Aanisah
Aanya
Aaralyn
Aaria
Aariana
Aarianna
Aaricia
Aariel
Aarielle
Aasia
Aava
Aayla
Ababuo
Abagail
Abaigael
Abaigeal
Abalina
Abana
Abarne
Abarrane
Abbatha
Abbetina
Abbey
Abbie
Abbigail
Abbigale

Abbott
Abby
Abcde
Abdera
Abebi
Abedabun
Abegail
Abegayle
Abeje
Abelia
Abelina
Abella
Abellona
Abena
Abeni
Abequa
Aberdeen
Aberfa
Abertha
Abetje
Abhirati
Abhy
Abia
Abiageal
Abiah
Abiba
Abichail
Abida
Abiela
Abigail
Abigale
Abigayle
Abihail
Abijah
Abila
Abilene
Abina
Abir
Abira
Abital
Abitha
Abla

Abra
Abree
Abri
Abrial
Abriana
Abrianna
Abrielle
Abrienda
Abrienne
Abril
Abt
Abyssinia
Acacia
Academia
Acadia
Acantha
Acasia
Accacia
Accalia
Aceline
Acelynn
Achava
Achazia
Achelle
Achinoam
Achsah
Acima
Acotas
Acquanetta
Acsah
Ad
Ada
Adabella
Adah
Adain
Adair
Adaira
Adairia
Adal
Adalbrechta
Adalene
Adalgisa

Adali
Adalia
Adalicia
Adalie
Adalina
Adaline
Adalira
Adaliz
Adallyn
Adalwolfa
Adalyn
Adalynn
Adamaris
Adamina
Adamma
Adana
Adanna
Adanya
Adar
Adara
Adasha
Adda
Addah
Addalyn
Addalynn
Addeline
Addfwyn
Addie
Addien
Addiena
Addilyn
Addison
Addisyn
Addriana
Addrianna
Addula
Addy
Addyson
Ade
Adecyn
Adeen
Adel

Adela
Adelaida
Adelaide
Adelajda
Adele
Adelee
Adeleh
Adelei
Adelheid
Adelheide
Adelia
Adelie
Adelina
Adelinda
Adelinde
Adeline
Adelisa
Adelise
Adelita
Adella
Adelle
Adellinde
Adelma
Adelpha
Adelphia
Adelyn
Adelynn
Adema
Ademia
Adena
Adene
Adenydd
Adeola
Aderes
Aderyn
Adesina
Adette
Adhara
Adhita
Adiba
Adie
Adiella

Adila
Adilene
Adilenne
Adima
Adin
Adina
Adinah
Adinam
Adine
Adira
Aditi
Adiva
Adlai
Adleida
Adlesha
Adleta
Adley
Admina
Adoette
Adolpha
Adolphine
Adoncia
Adonia
Adora
Adorabella
Adoracion
Adorlee
Adra
Adreana
Adreanna
Adria
Adrian
Adriana
Adriane
Adrianna
Adrianne
Adrie
Adrielle
Adrien
Adriene
Adrienna
Adrienne

63

Adrina	Agafia	Agramakova	Ailish	Akasha	Alary
Adsila	Agafiia	Agrata	Ailith	Akay	Alasa
Adva	Agafiya	Agripena	Ailsa	Akeelah	Alaska
Adviga	Agafokliia	Agripina	Ailsie	Akela	Alastair
Ady	Agafonika	Agrippa	Aim	Akemi	Alastrina
Adyna	Agafya	Agrippina	Aimara	Aki	Alastriona
Adyson	Agalia	Agueda	Aimee	Akia	Alathea
Aedon	Agape	Agyness	Aimée	Akibe	Alaula
Aegina	Agapi	Ahadi	Aimi	Akiha	Alaura
Aelan	Agapiia	Ahana	Aimilios	Akiko	Alavara
Aelfwine	Agasha	Aharona	Aina	Akilah	Alawa
Aeliana	Agashka	Ahava	Aindrea	Akili	Alayah
Aelrue	Agata	Ahave	Aine	Akilina	Alayja
Aelwen	Agate	Ahelie	Aingeal	Akillina	Alayna
Aelwyd	Agatha	Ahmoua	Aingealag	Akira	Alayne
Aelynthi	Agathe	Ahna	Ainhoa	Akiulina	Alaynna
Aenea	Agaton	Ahrendue	Aino	Akiva	Alaysia
Aeolia	Agaue	Ahskahala	Ainsley	Akosua	Alazne
Aerilaya	Agave	Ahuda	Ainslie	Aksana	Alba
Aerilyn	Agda	Ahuva	Aintzane	Aksinya	Albany
Aerin	Agdta	Ai	Air	Akuna	Albena
Aerith	Aggi	Aibhilin	Aira	Akyra	Alberga
Aero	Aggie	Aibhlin	Airi	Ala	Alberta
Aeron	Aghadreena	Aibhne	Airiana	Alaana	Alberte
Aerona	Aghamora	Aida	Airlea	Alabama	Albertina
Aeronwen	Aghaveagh	Aidan	Airlia	Alaglossa	Albertine
Aerwyna	Aghavilla	Aideen	Airlie	Alaia	Albertyne
Aeryn	Aghna	Aiden	Aisha	Alain	Albia
Aesara	Aglaia	Aidia	Aishwarya	Alaina	Albina
Aethelwyne	Aglaida	Aife	Aisley	Alaine	Albinia
Afaf	Aglauros	Aiglentina	Aislin	Alainna	Albinka
Afanasiia	Aglaya	Aigneis	Aisling	Alair	Albreda
Afanasiya	Agna	Aiken	Aislinn	Alais	Alcee
Afarin	Agnek	Aiko	Aisly	Alake	Alcestis
Affinity	Agnella	Aila	Aitana	Alala	Alchamy
Afia	Agnes	Ailana	Aithley	Alamea	Alchemy
Afifa	Agnese	Ailani	Aithne	Alameda	Alcie
Afimia	Agnessa	Ailat	Aitugan	Alana	Alcina
Afon	Agneta	Ailbhe	Aiya	Alandra	Alcinda
Afonaseva	Agnete	Aileana	Aiyana	Alane	Alcine
Afra	Agnetha	Aileen	Aiyanna	Alani	Alcinia
Afraima	Agnia	Aileene	Aizdiakova	Alanii	Alcott
Afric	Agniia	Ailey	Aizza	Alanis	Alcyone
Africa	Agnola	Aili	Aj	Alanna	Alcyoneus
Afrodille	Agotha	Ailia	Aja	Alannah	Alda
Afternoon	Agoti	Ailie	Ajua	Alanni	Aldeen
Afton	Agoyoanye	Ailin	Akako	Alannis	Alden
Afua	Agraciana	Ailis	Akane	Alanza	Aldene
Afya	Agrafena	Ailisa	Akantha	Alaqua	Aldina
Agacia	Agrafina	Ailise	Akari	Alarice	Aldis

Aldona	Alexandrea	Aliki	Allecra	Almarine	Altin
Aldonsa	Alexandria	Alile	Alleena	Almas	Alto
Aldonza	Alexandriana	Alima	Alleffra	Almeda	Alton
Aldora	Alexandrina	Alina	Allegra	Almera	Altsoba
Alea	Alexandrine	Alinae	Allegria	Almira	Alucia
Aleah	Alexane	Alinda	Allegro	Almithara	Aludra
Aleandra	Alexanndra	Aline	Allena	Almodine	Alufa
Aleccia	Alexcia	Alinna	Allene	Almond	Alula
Alecia	Alexi	Alisa	Allenna	Almudena	Aluma
Aleda	Alexia	Alisanne	Allete	Almunda	Alumina
Aledwen	Alexina	Alise	Allexa	Almundena	Alumit
Aleece	Alexine	Alisha	Allexandra	Almundina	Alura
Aleecia	Alexis	Alishia	Allexandria	Alodia	Alva
Aleela	Alexus	Alisia	Allexia	Alodie	Alvaerele
Aleena	Alexx	Alison	Allexis	Aloe	Alvah
Aleesha	Alexxa	Alissa	Alli	Aloha	Alvar
Aleeza	Alexxandra	Alissha	Allia	Alohi	Alvara
Aleezah	Alexxandria	Alisson	Allice	Alohilani	Alvarie
Alegra	Alexxia	Alisyn	Allicia	Aloisa	Alvarita
Alegria	Alexys	Alita	Allie	Aloise	Alvera
Aleid	Aleydis	Alithea	Allina	Aloisia	Alverdine
Aleigha	Alezae	Alitza	Allis	Aloma	Alverna
Alejandra	Alfhild	Alivette	Allisa	Alona	Alvina
Alejandrina	Alfonsa	Alivia	Allisha	Alondra	Alvita
Alek	Alfonsine	Alix	Allison	Alonna	Alvy
Aleka	Alfreda	Alixandra	Alliss	Alonsa	Alya
Aleksa	Algiana	Aliya	Allissa	Alonza	Alyanna
Aleksandra	Algoma	Aliyah	Allisson	Alora	Alyce
Alena	Alhambra	Aliyeh	Allisyn	Alouette	Alycia
Alene	Alhertina	Aliyn	Allivia	Alpana	Alyena
Alenka	Alhertine	Aliyya	Allona	Alpha	Alyenor
Alenna	Ali	Aliz	Allondra	Alphonsine	Alyn
Aleph	Alia	Aliza	Allonia	Alphonza	Alyna
Alera	Aliana	Alizabeth	Alloralla	Alphosine	Alyndra
Alerathla	Aliane	Alizah	Allsun	Alpina	Alyona
Aleshanee	Aliccia	Alize	Allura	Alpine	Alyra
Alesia	Alice	Alizée	Ally	Alsatia	Alys
Alessa	Alicen	Alizeh	Allyce	Alsie	Alysa
Alessandra	Alicia	Alizza	Allynna	Alta	Alyse
Alessia	Alicja	Alka	Allyriane	Altaf	Alysha
Alesta	Alick	Alkas	Allysa	Altagracia	Alyshea
Aleta	Alicyn	Alla	Allyse	Altair	Alyshia
Aletea	Alida	Allaina	Allysen	Altaira	Alysia
Aletha	Aliena	Allaire	Allysia	Altalune	Alyson
Alethea	Alienor	Allana	Allyson	Altantsetseg	Alyss
Aletia	Aliina	Allani	Allyssa	Alte	Alyssa
Aletta	Aliisa	Allannia	Allysse	Altessa	Alyssandra
Alex	Alijah	Allard	Allyssia	Althea	Alysse
Alexa	Alika	Allayna	Allysson	Altheda	Alyssia
Alexandra	Alikae	Allecia	Alma	Althia	Alysson

Alyvia	Amarah	Amethyst	Amoret	Analiese	Andi
Alzan	Amaranda	Ameya	Amorette	Analilia	Andie
Alzbet	Amarande	Amhi	Amori	Analisa	Andolina
Alzbeta	Amaranta	Ami	Amorica	Analise	Andorra
Alzea	Amarante	Amia	Amorie	Analisia	Andra
Alzena	Amarantha	Amiah	Amorina	Anamari	Andralyn
Alzina	Amaranthae	Amica	Amoris	Anamaria	Andrea
Ama	Amare	Amice	Amorita	Anamarie	Andreana
Amaani	Amari	Amidala	Amory	Anamika	Andree
Amabel	Amariah	Amie	Amoura	Anana	Andreea
Amabella	Amarilis	Amiee	Ampliia	Ananda	Andreeva
Amabelle	Amarilla	Amiel	Amra	Anang	Andreiana
Amabilis	Amarine	Amiela	Amrei	Anani	Andreina
Amable	Amaris	Amihan	Amrita	Ananta	Andren
Amada	Amarisa	Amii	Amser	Ananya	Andrina
Amadahy	Amarise	Amilia	Amy	Anara	Andria
Amadea	Amariss	Amina	Amya	Anarosa	Andrievicha
Amadi	Amarissa	Aminah	Amytis	Anarzee	Andromache
Amadika	Amarli	Aminali	Amzie	Anasazi	Andromeda
Amadine	Amarra	Aminia	An	Anastacia	Andy
Amadis	Amaryllis	Aminna	Ana	Anastasha	Ane
Amadore	Amata	Aminta	Anaaya	Anastasia	Anechka
Amai	Amaya	Amira	Anabel	Anastasiia	Aneirin
Amaia	Amayeta	Amirah	Anabell	Anastasija	Aneisha
Amaka	Ambar	Amisa	Anabella	Anastassia	Aneko
Amal	Amber	Amisquew	Anabelle	Anastazia	Anela
Amala	Amberlin	Amissa	Anacita	Anastazja	Anemone
Amalasanda	Amberly	Amit	Anaclaudia	Anat	Anemoon
Amalea	Ambika	Amita	Anael	Anata	Aneska
Amalfi	Ambra	Amite	Anaelle	Anatassia	Aneta
Amali	Ambre	Amitee	Anafa	Anate	Anetta
Amalia	Ambrea	Amithi	Anah	Anatie	Anette
Amalida	Ambrosia	Amitola	Anahella	Anatola	Anevay
Amalie	Ambrosine	Amity	Anahera	Anatolia	Anevy
Amalisa	Amedea	Amiya	Anahi	Anawrete	Anfiia
Amalthea	Amedee	Amiyah	Anahí	Anaxandra	Anfisa
Amalur	Amelfa	Amkissra	Anahid	Anaya	Anfoma
Amalure	Amelia	Amlaruil	Anahira	Anca	Anfusa
Amalya	Amelie	Amma	Anahita	Ance	Anga
Amana	Amélie	Ammanda	Anais	Ancelin	Ange
Amanda	Amelina	Ammara	Anaïs	Ancelina	Angel
Amandine	Amelinda	Ammber	Anakaren	Ancelote	Angela
Amandla	Ameline	Ammi	Anala	Anchoret	Angelea
Amani	Amellia	Ammiel	Analaura	Ancina	Angelee
Amanii	Amena	Ammy	Analee	Anda	Angelena
Amannda	America	Amna	Analeigh	Andeana	Angeletta
Amanni	Americus	Amnestria	Analena	Andena	Angelette
Amantha	Amerie	Amondi	AnaLeticia	Andera	Angeli
Amapola	Amery	Amor	Analia	Andere	Angelia
Amara	Ames	Amora	Analicia	Andes	Angelica

66

Angelie	Anisha	Annalisa	Annissa	Antonina	Aquaria
Angelika	Anisia	Annalise	Anniston	Antonnia	Aquarius
Angeliki	Anisiia	Annalisse	Annistyn	Anuhea	Aquene
Angelina	Anisiya	Annamaria	Annjelica	Anunciacion	Aquilia
Angeline	Anissa	Annamarie	Annmarie	Anusia	Aquilina
Angelinna	Anisya	Annastasia	Annona	Anwar	Aquinnah
Angelique	Anita	Annastasija	Annora	Anwen	Aquitaine
Angélique	Anitchka	Annastassia	Annorah	Anya	Aquitania
Angelisa	Anitia	Annaya	Annot	Anyssa	Ara
Angelita	Anitra	Anndra	Annsley	Anyuta	Arabela
Angell	Anitsa	Anndrea	Annunciata	Anyya	Arabele
Angella	Aniya	Anndria	Annuziata	Anzhela	Arabell
Angellia	Aniyah	AnnDrue	Annwyl	Anzu	Arabella
Angellica	Anizka	Anne	Anny	Aobh	Arabelle
Angellina	Anja	Anne Marie	Annya	Aoi	Arabesque
Angelou	Anjali	Anne-marie	Annze	Aoibh	Arabia
Angelynn	Anjanette	Anne-Marie	Anomie	Aoibhe	Araceli
Angeni	Anje	Anne-Will	Anona	Aoibheann	Aracelia
Anggie	Anjeanette	Anneke	Anonna	Aoibhinn	Aracelli
Angharad	Anjelica	Anneli	Anora	Aoife	Aracelly
Anghard	Anjelika	Anneliese	Anouck	Aoki	Aracely
Angie	Anjelita	Annelisa	Anouk	Aoko	Arachne
Angilia	Anjellica	Annelise	Anoush	Aolani	Aradia
Angusina	Anjie	Annemae	Anoushka	Aonani	Arafa
Angusta	Anjii	Annemarie	Anouska	Apala	Aram
Angyalka	Anjolie	Annemie	Ansa	Apfiia	Arama
Anhaern	Anju	Annemieke	Anselma	Aphra	Araminta
AnhDao	Anka	Annemarie	Ansleigh	Aphrodite	Araminte
Ani	Anke	Annerose	Ansley	Apirka	Aranga
Ania	Anki	Annesley	Ansonia	Apolinaria	Aranrhod
Anica	Ankti	Annette	Anstace	Apolinariia	Arantxa
Anice	Anku	Anngela	Anstice	Apollina	Arashel
Aniceta	Ann	Anngelica	Answer	Apolline	Araushnee
Anichka	Ann-Marie	Anngelina	Antalya	Apollonia	Arava
Aniela	Anna	Anngie	Anteia	Apollonis	Aravae
Anieli	Anna Maria	Annia	Anthea	Apoloniada	Aravis
Anielka	Anna Marie	Annica	Anthemia	Apolosakifa	Arawn
Anika	Annabel	Annice	Anthia	Apona	Araxie
Aniki	Annabella	Annick	Anticlea	Aponi	Arayna
Anikka	Annabell	Annie	Antigone	Apphia	Arbela
Aniko	Annabelle	Annik	Antiquity	Apple	Arbor
Anila	Annabeth	Annika	Antje	Apria	Arcade
Anima	Annabla	Annike	Antoinetta	April	Arcadia
Animaida	AnnaCristina	Annikka	Antoinette	Aprill	Arcaena
Animaisa	Annalee	Annikke	Antonella	Apsaras	Arcangela
Anina	Annaleigh	Annikki	Antonetta	Apulia	Arcelia
Aninda	Annali	Annily	Antonia	Aqila	Arcene
Anippe	Annalie	Annis	Antonidka	Aqua	Archana
Anisa	Annaliese	Annisa	Antonie	Aquamarine	Arcilla
Anise	Annalina	Annisha	Antonietta	Aquanetta	Arda

Ardala	Arianwen	Arlene	Artaith	Ashala	Asmara
Ardara	Arianwyn	Arlenis	Artemeva	Ashanti	Aspasia
Ardath	Aricela	Arlenne	Artemiia	Ashantii	Aspen
Arddun	Arich	Arlet	Artemis	Ashby	Asphodel
Ardea	Aricia	Arleta	Artemisia	Asheley	Aspyn
Ardeen	Aridatha	Arleth	Artemus	Ashely	Assa
Ardelis	Ariel	Arlette	Artha	Ashia	Assana
Ardelle	Ariela	Arley	Arthes	Ashira	Assane
Arden	Ariele	Arlinda	Arthuretta	Ashla	Assia
Ardice	Arielimnda	Arline	Arthurette	Ashlan	Assisi
Ardin	Ariella	Arlise	Arthurina	Ashland	Assunta
Ardis	Arielle	Arliss	Arthurine	Ashle	Asta
Ardith	Ariellel	Arlo	Artin	Ashlea	Astarte
Areille	Arien	Armanda	Artis	Ashlee	Aster
Areli	Aries	Armande	Artois	Ashleen	Astera
Arella	Arij	Armani	Artura	Ashleey	Asteria
Arelli	Arilla	Armantine	Aruna	Ashlei	Asthore
Arelly	Arin	Armel	Arunika	Ashleigh	Astin
Arely	Arina	Armelle	Arusha	Ashlen	Astolat
Aren	Arine	Armen	Arva	Ashley	Aston
Arena	Arion	Armena	Arverne	Ashli	Astoria
Arenda	Aris	Armenia	Arvid	Ashlie	Astra
Aretha	Arisa	Armes	Arwa	Ashliegh	Astraea
Arethusa	Arisha	Armida	Arwen	Ashlin	Astraia
Aretina	Arisje	Armina	Arwydd	Ashling	Astrea
Arevig	Arissa	Armona	Arya	Ashlley	Astred
Arezo	Arista	Arnalda	Aryan	Ashlly	Astri
Argel	Aristodeme	Arnarra	Aryana	Ashly	Astrid
Argene	Arius	Arnelle	Aryann	Ashlyn	Astrithr
Argenta	Ariya	Arnette	Aryanna	Ashlynn	Astynome
Argentia	Ariyah	Arnia	Arza	Ashlynne	Asuka
Argentina	Ariyne	Arnina	Asa	Ashni	Asuncion
Argia	Ariza	Arnola	Asabi	Ashra	Asya
Arglwyddes	Arizona	Arnon	Asaka	Ashten	Atahladte
Argoel	Arjean	Aroa	Asali	Ashtin	Atalanta
Argraff	Arkadina	Aroha	Asami	Ashton	Atalaya
Ari	Arkansas	Aroha	Asante	Ashtyn	Atalia
Aria	Arketah	Arooj	Asasia	Ashtynn	Atalie
Ariadna	Arkhipa	Arorangi	Asatira	Ashwini	Atalya
Ariadne	Arkhippa	Arpina	Ascella	Asia	Atara
Ariah	Arla	Arrayah	Ascencion	Asiah	Atarah
Arial	Arlais	Arria	Asela	Asianah	Ataret
Arian	Arlana	Arrian	Asemina	Asima	Atepa
Ariana	Arlanna	Arriana	Asenath	Asis	Atera
Ariane	Arlayna	Arrianna	Asencion	Asisa	Ateret
Arianell	Arleana	Arriel	Asenka	Askitreia	Atgas
Arianna	Arleen	Arriell	Asenke	Askitriia	Athaleyah
Arianne	Arleene	Arrietty	Asgre	Asli	Athalia
Arianrhod	Arleigh	Arsenia	Ash	Asma	Athalie
Arianthe	Arlena	Arsinoe	Asha	Asmaa	Athanasia

68

Athdara	Audrey Maud	Austynn	Avita	Ayira	Azul	
Atheena	Audrey Maude	Autonoe	Avital	Ayishah	Azura	
Athelas	Audria	Auttumn	Aviva	Ayita	Azure	
Athena	Audriana	Autumn	Avivah	Ayla		
Atherton	Audrianna	Autumnn	Avivi	Ayleen	## B	
Athiambo	Audrie	Ava	Avivit	Aylin		
Athracht	Audrielle	Avaani	Aviya	Aylla	Baara	
Atia	Audrina	Avagail	Avon	Ayn	Baba	
Atifa	Audrinna	Avah	Avonaco	Ayo	Babe	
Atira	Audris	Avalbane	Avongara	Ayoka	Babette	
Atiya	Audry	Avaline	Avonlea	Aysel	Babita	
Atl	August	Avalon	Avonmora	Aysha	Baby	
Atlanta	Augusta	Avalyn	Avramova	Aysia	BachYen	
Atlantis	Augusteen	Avani	Avril	Ayu	Baden	
Atlee	Augustina	Avanni	Avrill	Ayuka	Bader	
Atoosa	Augustine	Avari	Avva	Ayume	Badr	
Atria	Auina	Avariella	Avye	Ayumi	Badu	
Atropos	Aulani	Avarielle	Aweinon	Ayumu	Baez	
Atsuko	Aulii	Avatari	Awel	Ayunli	Baha	
Atthis	Aulis	Avdeeva	Awen	Aza	Bahaar	
Attilia	Auluua	Avdiushka	Awena	Azabeth	Bahati	
Auberon	Aundrea	Avdotia	Awenasa	Azalea	Bahia	
Auberta	Aura	Ave	Awendea	Azalee	Bahira	
Aubina	Aurae	Aveline	Awendela	Azalia	Bai	
Aubine	Auralee	Avelyn	Awenita	Azam	Baia	
Aubrecia	Aure	Aven	Awentia	Azami	Baialyn	
Aubree	Aurel	Avena	Awinita	Azana	Baibichia	
Aubrey	Aurelia	Avera	Axelia	Azania	Baibre	
Aubri	Aureliana	Averi	Axella	Azar	Baila	
Aubriana	Aurelie	Averie	Axelle	Azarel	Bailee	
Aubrianna	Auren	Averil	Axilya	Azaria	Baileigh	
Aubrianne	Aurex	Averill	Axl	Azariah	Bailey	
Aubrie	Auria	Averna	Aya	Azelia	Baili	
Aubriee	Aurica	Avery	Ayaana	Azelie	Bailie	
Aubrielle	Auriel	Avgusta	Ayaka	Azenor	Bailley	
Auburn	Aurielle	Avi	Ayako	Azha	Baillie	
Aud	Aurinda	Avia	Ayala	Azhar	Baily	
Auda	Aurkena	Avian	Ayalah	Azia	Baina	
Aude	Aurkene	Aviana	Ayame	Aziel	Bairbre	
Auden	Aurnia	Avianna	Ayami	Aziza	Baize	
Audene	Aurora	Avice	Ayana	Azize	Baja	
Audey	Aurorette	Avichayil	Ayane	Azmina	Baka	
Audi	Aurum	Avidan	Ayanna	Azni	Baker	
Audra	Auryon	Aviela	Ayano	Azra	Bakhteiarova	
Audrea	Auset	Avigail	Ayasha	Azriel	Bakura	
Audreanne	Austen	Avignon	Ayashe	Azu	Bala	
Audree	Austin	Avila	Ayda	Azuba	Balbara	
Audrey	Austine	Avinoam	Ayeesha	Azubah	Balbina	
Audrey Ann	Australia	Avis	Ayelet	Azucena	Baldwin	
Audrey Anne	Austria	Avisa	Ayesha	Azuka	Baleigh	

Bali	Bat	Becka	Belukha	Berniss	Betje
Ballade	Batel	Beckett	Belva	Bernita	Betrys
Ballari	Bates	Becky	Bem	Bernyce	Betsan
Ballencia	Bathilda	Beda	Bena	Berry	Betsey
Ballou	Bathsheba	Bedche	Benecia	Bert	Betsy
Bambalina	Bathshira	Bede	Benedetta	Berta	Betta
Bambi	Batsheva	Bedegraine	Benedicta	Berth	Bette
Bambina	Battista	Bedelia	Bengta	Bertha	Betti
Banana	Battseeyon	Bee	Benicia	Berthe	Bettina
Bandana	Battzion	Beecher	Benigna	Berthog	Bettine
Bane	Batu	Beeja	Benilde	Berti	Bettsy
Banee	Batya	Begonia	Benita	Bertilde	Betty
Banji	Bay	Begum	Benjamina	Bertille	Beula
Banks	Baya	Behati	Benka	Bertina	Beulah
Banner	Bayan	Behira	Bennett	Bertrade	Bev
Banon	Bayarmaa	Behitha	Bennington	Bertrice	Beverley
Bao	Bayle	Beibhinn	Benoite	Bertrona	Beverly
Baptista	Baylea	Beige	Bente	Bertrun	Bevin
Bara	Bayleah	Bel	Bentley	Berura	Beyla
Baraka	Baylee	Bela	Beonica	Beruria	Beyonce
Barb	Bayleigh	Belanna	Bera	Beruriah	Beyoncé
Barbara	Bayley	Belda	Beracha	Beryl	Beyoncee
Barbaraa	Bayli	Beleka	Berangaria	Bess	Bezruchka
Barbie	Baylie	Belen	Berdina	Bessie	Bezubaia
Barbina	Baylor	Belén	Berdine	Beta	Bezui
Barbra	Bayo	Belgis	Berengaria	Betelgeuse	Bhavna
Barbro	Bayou	Belgukovna	Berenice	Beth	Bhudevi
Barcelona	Bazhena	Belia	Beres	Betha	Bian
Bardot	Bea	Belicia	Beretta	Bethan	Biana
Bariah	Beagan	Belinda	Bergen	Bethanee	Bianca
Barinda	Beah	Beline	Bergitta	Bethani	Biancca
Barr	Bean	Belisma	Berit	Bethania	Bianka
Barra	Beata	Belita	Berkeley	Bethanie	Biannca
Barran	Beate	Belka	Berlynn	Bethann	Biata
Barras	Beatha	Bell	Bermuda	Bethannie	Bibi
Barrett	Beathag	Bella	Bern	Bethanny	Bibiana
Barrie	Beathas	Bellachay	Bernadea	Bethany	Bibiane
Barry	Beatrice	Belladonna	Bernadette	Bethari	Bibishkina
Bartha	Beatrisa	Bellamy	Bernadina	Bethea	Bibsbebe
Barunka	Beatrix	Bellanca	Bernadine	Bethel	Bice
Baruska	Beatriz	Bellance	Bernarda	Betheli	Bich
Basanti	Beauty	Bellatrix	Berne	Bethenny	Bichette
Basha	Bebba	Belle	Berneen	Bethesda	Bidaban
Basia	Bebe	Bellerose	Bernelle	Bethia	Biddy
Basilia	Bebhinn	Bellezza	Bernetta	Bethoc	Bidelia
Basima	Becca	Bellinda	Bernette	Bethsaida	Bidina
Basira	Bechet	Bellini	Berni	Bethseda	Bidu
Basma	Bechette	Bellissa	Bernice	Bethsheba	Bienna
Basmat	Bechira	Bellona	Bernicia	Bethune	Bienne
Bastet	Beck	Beloved	Bernique	Bethwyn	Bienvenida

Bifrost	Blanca	Bogdana	Bozi	Brayne	Brianne
Biiata	Blanch	Bogna	Bozica	Brazil	Briar
Bijou	Blanche	Bogukhvala	Braceletto	Bre	Brice
Bijoux	Blanchefleur	Bogumezt	Bracha	Brea	Bricen
Bikita	Blanda	Bogumila	Brachah	Breahna	Brid
Bilge	Blandina	Boguslava	Bracken	Breana	Bride
Bilhah	Blanka	Bohdana	Bradana	Breandan	Bridge
Biljana	Blanket	Boheme	Braddock	Breann	Bridget
Billa	Blaque	Bohemia	Bradley	Breanna	Bridgett
Billi	Blasa	Bohgana	Brady	Breanne	Bridgette
Billie	Blasia	Bohumile	Bradyn	Brechtje	Bridgit
Billy	Blathnat	Boika	Brae	Breck	Bridie
Bimala	Blausa	Boinedal	Braeden	Breckin	Brie
Bina	Blaze	Bolade	Braelyn	Breda	Briella
Binah	Blenda	Bolanile	Braelynn	Brede	Brielle
Binda	Blessing	Bolanle	Braerindra	Bree	Brienda
Binder	Blessy	Bolbe	Braewyn	Breea	Brienna
Bindi	Bleu	Bolce	Bragina	Breeda	Brienne
Binge	Blima	Boldina	Braith	Breen	Brier
Binney	Blimah	Bolemila	Brande	Breena	Brigantia
Binnie	Bliss	Boleslava	Brandee	Breeze	Brigetta
Binta	Blissany	Bolgarina	Brandi	Breezy	Brigette
Binyamina	Blithe	Bolgarynia	Brandice	Bregus	Brighid
Bionda	Bliths	Bolivia	Brandie	Breindel	Brighton
Bird	Blix	Bolormaa	Brandii	Brencis	Brigid
Birdena	Blodwedd	Bona	Brandilyn	Brenda	Brigida
Birdie	Blodwen	Bonanza	Brandissa	Brendaa	Brigidia
Birdy	Blodwyn	Bonfilia	Brandy	Brendalynn	Brigidine
Birgit	Bloem	Bonita	Brandye	Brendolyn	Brigit
Birgitta	Blondell	Bonnalurie	Brangwen	Brendy	Brigitta
Biriuta	Blondelle	Bonni	Brangwy	Brenna	Brigitte
Bisa	Blondene	Bonnie	Branice	Brennan	Brilane
Bisma	Blondie	Bonny	Branislava	Brennda	Brileigh
Bithron	Bloodrayne	Bonny-jean	Branizlawa	Brenta	Briley
Bithynia	Blossom	Bonny-lee	Branka	Brentley	Brilie
Bitsy	Blue	Boo	Brann	Breonna	Brillana
Bituin	Bluebell	Bora	Brantley	Bret	Brilliant
Bitya	Bluma	Borbala	Branwen	Brett	Brina
Bizzy	Bly	Borghild	Branwenn	Bretta	Brinda
Bjork	Blyana	Borisova	Branwyn	Brettany	Brinkley
Blainc	Blysse	Boriuta	Branxton	Brette	Brinley
Blair	Blythe	Borka	Brasen	Brevyn	Brinly
Blaire	Blythswana	Borsala	Brasilia	Bria	Brinsley
Blaise	Bo	Botilda	Bratomila	Brial	Brinti
Blake	Boadicea	Boudicca	Bratromila	Briallan	Brintie
Blakeley	Bobbi	Bouvier	Bratrumila	Briallen	Brio
Blakely	Bobbie	Boyana	Braulia	Briana	Briona
Blakeney	Bobby	Bozena	Brayden	Brianda	Brionna
Blakesleigh	Bodgana	Bozhana	Braylee	Brianna	Briony
Blakesley	Bodie	Bozhitsa	Braylin	Briannah	Brisa

Briseis	Brogan	Bryttany	Cadencia	Caitrin	Callisto
Brisha	Bron	Bryttni	Cadenza	Caitriona	Callula
Brisia	Brona	Buana	Cadette	Cal	Calpurnia
Brissa	Bronach	Buddug	Cadha	Cala	Caltha
Bristol	Bronislava	Budisla	Cadhla	Calais	Calvina
Brit	Bronnen	Budizla	Cadi	Calamity	Calvine
Brita	Bronte	Budshka	Cadie	Calandra	Calynda
Britain	Brontee	Budska	Cadwyn	Calandre	Calynn
Britaney	Bronwen	Buena	Cady	Calandria	Calypso
Britani	Bronwyn	Buenaventura	Cadyna	Calantha	Calysta
Britanie	Bronwynn	Buffy	Cael	Calanthe	Cam
Britannia	Bronx	Bukhval	Caela	Calarel	Camber
Britanny	Bronya	Bulan	Caelan	Calder	Cambree
Britany	Brook	Bulana	Caerthynna	Caldwell	Cambria
Brite	Brooke	Bunme	Caerwyn	Caledon	Cambrie
Brites	Brooklee	Bunny	Caesarea	Caledonia	Camden
Britin	Brooklyn	Bunty	Caethes	Calee	Camdyn
British	Brooklynn	Buona	Cafell	Caleigh	Camelia
Britnee	Brooklynne	Burgandy	Caffara	Calendre	Camellia
Britney	Brooks	Burgundy	Caffaria	Caley	Cameo
Britnie	Brucie	Burma	Cage	Calgary	Camera
Britny	Bruna	Burnett	Cagney	Cali	Cameron
Britt	Brunella	Burrell	Cahira	Caliana	Camila
Britta	Brunetta	Bushra	Cahya	Calico	Camile
Brittanee	Brunhild	Busy	Cai	Calida	Camilla
Brittaney	Brunhilda	Butch	Caia	California	Camille
Brittani	Brunonia	Buthainah	Caieta	Calina	Camillei
Brittania	Bruriah	Butrus	Cailean	Calinda	Camisha
Brittanie	Bryana	Buttercup	Caileigh	Calissa	Camishia
Brittanny	Bryanna	Butterfly	Cailin	Calista	Cammeo
Brittany	Bryanne	Byanca	Cailleach	Calixta	Cammi
Britten	Bryce	Byrd	Caillic	Calixte	Campana
Britteny	Brycin	Byrdie	Caily	Calla	Campbell
Brittiany	Brye		Cailyn	Callaghan	Camryn
Brittin	Brygid	**C**	Caimbrie	Callahan	Canada
Brittini	Brygida		Cain	Callan	Canan
Brittiny	Brylee	Cabalina	Cairistiona	Callas	Canary
Brittnay	Bryleigh	Cable	Cairo	Calle	Candace
Brittnee	Brylie	Caca	Cais	Callee	Candela
Brittney	Bryn	Cacey	Cait	Calleigh	Candelaria
Brittni	Bryna	Cache	Caitie	Callen	Candi
Brittnie	Brynda	Cachet	Caitilin	Calli	Candia
Brittny	Bryndis	Cacia	Caitir	Callia	Candice
Britton	Brynja	Cactus	Caitlyn	Callias	Candid
Brittony	Brynlee	Cade	Caitlan	Callidora	Candida
Britttany	Brynn	Cadeau	Caitland	Callie	Candide
Briza	Brynna	Cadee	Caitlin	Calligenia	Candie
Brocky	Bryony	Cadelaria	Caitlinn	Calliope	Candis
Brodie	Bryssa	Caden	Caitlyn	Callison	Candiss
Brody	Bryttani	Cadence	Caitlynn	Callista	Candra

72

Candy	Carin	Carnation	Casey	Cathy	Ceinlys
Cane	Carina	Carney	Cashlin	Catia	Ceinwen
Caneadea	Carine	Caro	Cashmere	Catie	Ceira
Canens	Carinna	Carol	Casidhe	Catina	Ceire
Caniad	Carinthia	Carola	Casilda	Catlee	Ceirios
Canika	Carisa	Carolan	Casiphia	Catlin	Cela
Canna	Carissa	Carole	Cass	Catline	Celaeno
Cannan	Carita	Carolena	Cassandan	Catlyn	Celandia
Cannelita	Caritas	Carolina	Cassandra	Cato	Celandine
Canta	Carla	Caroline	Cassandrea	Caton	Cele
Cantara	Carlee	Carolline	Cassara	Catori	Celeena
Cantata	Carleen	Carollyn	Cassee	Catreen	Celena
Cantrelle	Carleigh	Carollynn	Cassi	Catrice	Celene
Canyon	Carleigha	Carolyn	Cassia	Catrin	Celerina
Caoilainn	Carlen	Carolyne	Cassiane	Catrina	Celesse
Caoilfhionn	Carlena	Carolynn	Cassidy	Catrine	Celesta
Caoimhe	Carlene	Caron	Cassie	Catrinetta	Celeste
Caparina	Carletta	Carona	Cassiopeia	Catrinette	Celestia
Capella	Carley	Carondelet	Cassondra	Catrinia	Celestiel
Cappella	Carli	Caroun	Casta	Catriona	Celestina
Capri	Carlie	Carra	Castalia	Catryn	Celestine
Caprice	Carlijn	Carressa	Castel	Cattee	Celestte
Capricorn	Carlin	Carri	Castiel	Cavana	Celestyn
Capta	Carlina	Carrie	Cat	Cavanaugh	Celestyna
Capucina	Carling	Carrieann	Cataleya	Cawny	Celia
Capucine	Carlisle	Carrigan	Cataleyah	Caycee	Celie
Cara	Carlita	Carrina	Catalin	Cayenne	Celina
Carabella	Carlla	Carrington	Catalina	Cayla	Celinda
Carabelle	Carlota	Carrola	Catalyn	Caylee	Celine
Caraf	Carlotta	Carroll	Catarina	Cayleen	Celinna
Caraid	Carly	Carrolyn	Catarine	Cayley	Cella
Caralisa	Carlyle	Carryn	Cate	Caylie	Celleste
Caralyn	Carlyn	Carson	Cateline	Caylin	Cellia
Caralynn	Carlynda	Carsyn	Catelyn	Ceallach	Cellina
Carbry	Carman	Carter	Caterina	Ceana	Celosia
Cardea	Carmel	Carwen	Cath	Ceara	Celsey
Carden	Carmela	Cary	Catharine	Cece	Celyn
Careen	Carmelina	Carya	Cathasach	Cecelia	Cendrillon
Carella	Carmeline	Caryl	Cathay	Cecellia	Cendrine
Carelyn	Carmelita	Caryn	Catherin	Cecile	Cenedra
Caress	Carmella	Carynn	Catherine	Cecilia	Cenobia
Carcssa	Carmcn	Carys	Cathcryn	Cccillc	Ccrclia
Caresse	Carmencita	Caryss	Catheryna	Cecillia	Ceres
Carey	Carmiela	Casandra	Cathie	Cecilly	Cerese
Cari	Carmilla	Cascada	Cathlyn	Cecily	Ceri
Cariad	Carmina	Cascade	Cathleen	Cecislava	Ceria
Cariana	Carminda	Cascadia	Cathlin	Cedar	Ceridwen
Caridad	Carmindy	Cascata	Cathrine	Cedrica	Cerise
Carilla	Carmita	Case	Cathryn	Ceil	Cersei
Carilyn	Carna	Casee	Cathrynn	Ceilidh	Cerulean

73

Cerulia	Chandra	Charisma	Chasina	Chelssy	Cheryl
Cerys	Chandrelle	Chariss	Chasity	Chelsy	Cheryll
Cesara	Chanel	Charissa	Chassidy	Chemislava	Cheryth
Cesaria	Chanell	Charisse	Chastity	Chen	Chesa
Cesarina	Chanelle	Charita	Chasya	Chenelle	Chesislava
Cesia	Chaney	Charity	Chauncey	Chenille	Chesleigh
Cessair	Change	Charla	Chaundra	Chenka	Chesna
Ceteria	Chanina	Charlaine	Chaunte	Chenoa	Chesney
Ceyla	Chaniya	Charlayne	Chauntel	Chephtziba	Chess
Ceylon	Chanlyeya	Charlee	Chava	Chephzibah	Chessa
Cezanne	Channah	Charleen	Chavazelet	Chepi	Chessie
Cha'kwaina	Channary	Charleena	Chavela	Chepzibah	Chetanzi
Chaba	Channel	Charleene	Chavelle	Cher	Chevelle
Chabah	Channell	Charleigh	Chavi	Chere	Chevis
Chabela	Channelle	Charlena	Chaviva	Cheree	Chevonne
Chabelly	Channer	Charlene	Chavive	Chereen	Cheyanna
Chabely	Channery	Charlesetta	Chay	Cherell	Cheyanne
Chablis	Channing	Charleston	Chaya	Cherelle	Cheyenne
Chaela	Channon	Charlette	Chayele	Cherene	Cheyne
Chaeli	Chanson	Charley	Chayka	Cheri	Chezarina
Chaenath	Chantae	Charli	Chayla	Cherice	Chiaki
Chaggit	Chantal	Charlie	Chaylea	Cherida	Chiana
Chahna	Chantall	Charliee	Chaylse	Cherie	Chianna
Chaia	Chantalle	Charlii	Chazona	Cherilyn	Chiara
Chailyn	Chantay	Charline	Chebotova	Cherina	Chiarra
Chainey	Chante	Charlisa	Cheche	Cherine	Chica
Chaka	Chantel	Charlita	Chedva	Cherise	Chicago
Chakaluka	Chantell	Charlize	Cheena	Cherish	Chick
Chakra	Chantelle	Charlot	Chekhina	Cherisse	Chickoa
Chalice	Chanter	Charlotta	Chekhyna	Cherita	Chiharu
Chalina	Chantesuta	Charlotte	Chela	Cherith	Chihiro
Chalondra	Chanteyukan	Charly	Chelan	Cherlin	Chiho
Chalsarda	Chantilly	Charlyn	Chelby	Chermona	Chika
Chalsie	Chanton	Charmain	Chelci	Chernavka	Chikage
Chamania	Chantoya	Charmaine	Chelcie	Chernislava	Chikako
Chamayra	Chantrea	Charmayne	Cheliadina	Chernka	Chiku
Chambray	Chantrell	Charmian	Chelle	Cherokee	Chilam
Chameli	Chantry	Charmine	Chelley	Cherree	Chilli
Chamois	Chanya	Charna	Chellsea	Cherrell	Chimalis
Chamomile	Chao	Charnell	Chellsey	Cherrelle	Chimalus
Chamonix	Chapa	Charo	Chellsie	Cherri	Chimere
Chamutal	Chapin	Charra	Chelsa	Cherrie	Chimislava
Chan	Chappell	Charty	Chelse	Cherrill	China
Chana	Chara	Charumati	Chelsea	Cherris	Chinara
Chanah	Charae	Charybdis	Chelsee	Cherrise	Chinatsu
Chancee	Chardae	Chas	Chelsey	Cherrish	Chinna
Chanda	Chardon	Chasen	Chelsi	Cherrisse	Chinue
Chandana	Chardonnay	Chasiah	Chelsia	Cherry	Chiona
Chandelle	Charee	Chasianna	Chelsie	Cherryl	Chione
Chandler	Charis	Chasidah	Chelssie	Cherryll	Chipo

Chiqueta	Christianna	Cinzia	Cleantha	Codee	Conchobara
Chiquita	Christie	Cionnaye	Clelia	Codi	Conchobarra
Chiquitta	Christina	Cipriana	Clemance	Cody	Conchobarre
Chisuzu	Christine	Ciqala	Clematis	Coe	Concordia
Chita	Christmas	Cira	Clemence	Coeur	Condoleeza
Chitrinee	Christo	Circe	Clemencia	Coira	Condoleezza
Chitsa	Christobel	Ciri	Clemency	Colandra	Cong
Chiudka	Christy	Cirila	Clemensia	Colbie	Congalie
Chiyo	Chroma	Cissy	Clementina	Colby	Connal
Chiyoko	Chrysann	Cithara	Clementine	Colee	Connecticut
Chizue	Chrysantha	Citlali	Cleo	Coleka	Connelly
Chlo	Chrysanthe	Citlalli	Cleone	Colene	Connemara
Chloe	Chrysanthemum	Citra	Cleonie	Coleta	Connery
Chloris	Chryseis	Citron	Cleopatra	Coletta	Connie
Cho	Chrystal	Clymene	Cleora	Colette	Connolly
Chobotova	Chrystina	Ciyradyl	Cleta	Coligny	Connor
Chochmingwu	Chulda	Clair	Cleva	Colina	Connstance
Chofa	Chuma	Claire	Clever	Coline	Conradine
Choire	Chumani	Clancy	Clia	Colissa	Conshita
Chole	Chyna	Clara	Cliantha	Colista	Consolacion
Cholena	Chynica	Clarabelle	Clidhna	Colleen	Consolata
Chomylla	Chynna	Claral	Clio	Collena	Consolation
Chorine	Chyse	Claramae	Cliona	Collene	Constance
Chosovi	Cia	Clare	Clodagh	Colletta	Constancia
Chosposi	Ciana	Claret	Clodia	Collette	Constansie
Chou	Cianna	Clareta	Clodovea	Collice	Constantia
Chouko	Ciara	Clarette	Clor	Collins	Constantina
Chrina	Ciatlllait	Claribel	Cloria	Collis	Constanza
Chris	Cicada	Clarice	Clorinda	Colmcilla	Constanze
Chrisanna	Cicely	Clariee	Cloris	Colombia	Constanzie
Chrisanne	Cicilia	Clarimond	Clothilde	Colombine	Consuela
Chriselda	Cicily	Clarimonde	Clotho	Colony	Consuello
Chrishauna	Ciel	Clarinda	Clotilda	Colorado	Consuelo
Chrissa	Cielo	Clarion	Cloud	Columba	Content
Chrissie	Ciera	Clarisa	Cloudy	Columbia	Contessa
Chrissy	Ciernislava	Clariss	Clove	Columbine	Cookie
Christa	Cierra	Clarissa	Clover	Colwyn	Cooper
Christabel	Cili	Clarissant	Clovia	Comet	Copper
Christal	Cilia	Clarisse	Cluny	Comfort	Cora
Christana	Cilicia	Clarita	Clymene	Comforte	Coral
Christeen	Cilivren	Clarity	Clytie	Como	Coralee
Christel	Cilla	Claude	Coahoma	Comsuelo	Coralia
Christelle	Cimarron	Claudette	Coaxoch	comter	Coralie
Christen	Cimmaron	Claudia	Cobalt	Comyna	Coraline
Christena	Cinda	Claudie	Coby	Conary	Coraly
Christi	Cinder	Claudina	Cochava	Concepcion	Corazana
Christia	Cinderella	Claudine	Cocheta	Concepta	Corazon
Christian	Cindy	Clavdia	Cochise	Concetta	Corbeau
Christiana	Cinnabar	Clayne	Coco	Conchetta	Corbin
Christiane	Cinnamon	Clea	Cocoa	Conchita	Corby

Cordelia	Cosimia	Cristyn	Cyprian	Daira	Dana
Cordis	Cosma	Crosby	Cypris	Daisey	Danae
Cordula	Costa	Crotilda	Cyprus	Daisi	Danah
Coreen	Cotovatre	Cruella	Cyra	Daissy	Danaye
Coreene	Cotton	Cruise	Cyrah	Daisy	Dancer
Corentine	Coty	Cruz	Cyrene	Daja	Dane
Coretta	Countess	Cruzita	Cyrilla	Dakira	Danea
Corette	Courtenay	Crwys	Cyrille	Dakota	Danee
Corey	Courteney	Crysta	Cyrillia	Dalal	Danele
Cori	Courtline	Crystal	Cytherea	Dale	Danelea
Coriander	Courtlyn	Crystall	Cytheria	Dalee	Danelle
Coriann	Courtnee	Csilla	Cyzarine	Dalena	Danesha
Corianne	Courtnei	Cualli	Czarina	Dalenna	Danessa
Corie	Courtney	Cuba	Czeimislawa	Daleyza	Danette
Corin	Courtni	Cullodena		Dalia	Dangela
Corina	Courtnie	Cullodina	**D**	Daliah	Dangelis
Corine	Courtny	Cumania		Dalida	Dani
Corinna	Coy	Cumina		Dalila	Dania
Corinne	Coye	Cundrie	D'arcy	Dalilah	Danica
Corinthia	Cragen	Cunnawabum	Da-xia	Dalileh	Daniela
Corisa	Crane	Curran	Daana	Dalili	Daniella
Corisande	Crecia	Curry	Daania	Dalinda	Danielle
Corissa	Creda	Curtis	Daba	Dalis	Danifa
Corliss	Cree	Cushla	Dabney	Dalisay	Danika
Cornelia	Creiddylad	Cuthberta	Dacey	Dalit	Danikka
Cornella	Creissant	Cwen	Dacia	Daliunda	Danila
Coro	Creola	Cyan	Dada	Daliyah	Danilova
Corona	Crescent	Cyane	Dae	Dallas	Danique
Coronis	Crescentia	Cyanea	Dael	Dallis	Danit
Corra	Cressida	Cyanne	Daelyn	Dallon	Danita
Correen	Crete	Cybele	Daena	Dally	Daniyah
Correena	Cricket	Cybil	Daenerys	Dallyce	Danna
Corri	Crimson	Cybill	Daere	Dalmace	Dannee
Corrianna	Crisann	Cybille	Daeva	Dama	Dannell
Corrianne	Crisanna	Cyd	Daffodil	Damali	Dannelle
Corrie	Crisanta	Cyder	Dafna	Damalis	Danni
Corrina	Crispina	Cydney	Dafne	Damani	Dannia
Corrine	Crissa	Cylia	Dagan	Damara	Dannica
Corry	Crissie	Cyma	Daganya	Damaris	Danniela
Corsen	Crissy	Cymbeline	Daganyah	Damariss	Danniell
Corsica	Crista	Cymreiges	Dagmar	Damayanti	Danniella
Cortnee	Cristal	Cynara	Dagny	Dameka	Dannielle
Cortney	Cristeen	Cyndi	Dahl	Damia	Dannika
Cortni	Cristen	Cynna	Dahlia	Damiana	Dannon
Cortnie	Cristi	Cynnthia	Dahliana	Damiane	Danny
Corvina	Cristie	Cynthia	Dahna	Damica	Dantea
Corwin	Cristin	Cynthiaa	Dahnya	Damien	Danu
Cory	Cristina	Cyntia	Dai	Damita	Danube
Cosette	Cristine	Cynzia	Daija	Damla	Dany
Cosima	Cristy	Cypress	Daijah	Damonica	Danya
			Daina		

76

Danyale	Darnell	Dawn	Decembra	Delfina	Demia
Danylynn	Darnetta	Dawna	Decima	Delia	Demidova
Daphna	Darnisha	Dawndrell	Decla	Delicah	Demii
Daphnah	Daromila	Dawnn	Deda	Délice	Demmi
Daphne	Daron	Day	Dedenia	Delicia	Democracy
Daphnee	Darra	Daya	Dedre	Deliciae	Dena
Dara	Darrah	Dayaa	Dee	Delight	Denae
Daracha	Darrell	Dayami	Deeana	Delila	Denali
Darah	Darren	Dayana	Deeandra	Delilah	Denay
Daralis	Darria	Dayanara	Deeann	Delimbiyra	Denelle
Daratrine	Darsha	Dayannara	Deeanna	Delisa	Denequa
Daray	Darshee	Dayla	DeeDee	Delise	Deni
Darby	Daru	Daylann	Deedra	Delisha	Denia
Darcel	Daruka	Dayle	Deelilah	Delit	Denica
Darcell	Darva	Dayleen	Deena	Deliz	Denice
Darcelle	Darya	Daylin	Deenna	Delja	Denicha
Darcey	Daryl	Dayna	Deepnita	Dell	Denicia
Darchelle	Daryn	Dayo	Deetra	Della	Deniece
Darci	Dash	Daysi	Dehateh	Dellaney	Denim
Darcia	Dasha	Dayton	Deianira	Dellen	Denisa
Darcie	Dashania	Daytona	Deidra	Dellia	Denise
Darcy	Dashawna	Dea	Deidre	Delling	Denisha
Darda	Dasia	Deah	Deidree	Delma	Denissa
Dareen	Dasyra	Dean	Deiene	Delmar	Denisse
Darena	Datherine	Deana	Deifilia	Delmara	Denita
Darerca	Dathlue	Deandra	Deikun	Delmare	Deniz
Dargiana	Datja	Deane	Deina	Delmira	Denna
Dari	Datya	Deann	Deiondra	Delora	Dennise
Daria	Datyah	Deanna	Deiondre	Delores	Dennisse
Darian	Daughtry	Deanndra	Deirdra	Delphi	Denny
Dariann	Dava	Deanne	Deirdre	Delphia	Denver
Darice	Davan	Dearbhail	Deisy	Delphina	Denyse
Dariel	Daveigh	Deasia	Deitra	Delphine	Deolinda
Dariela	Daveney	Debbie	Deja	Delshandra	Deon
Darielle	Davi	Debborah	Déja	Delsie	Deona
Darien	Davida	Debborrah	Dejaa	Delta	Deondra
Darina	Davignon	Debbra	Dejanae	Deltha	Deonn
Darissa	Davin	Debby	Deka	Delu	Deonna
Daritsa	Davina	Debonnaire	Dekava	Delwyn	Deonne
Darja	Davinah	Debora	Dekedrian	Delyth	Deora
Dark	Davine	Deboraah	Dekhova	Demanda	Dera
Darla	Davinia	Deborah	Del	Demarius	Derby
Darleena	Davinna	Deborahh	delaida	Demas	Deretka
Darleene	Davitah	Deborrah	Delaine	Dembe	Derforgal
Darlena	Davite	Debra	Delaire	Demelza	Derforgala
Darlene	Davonna	Debrah	Delana	Dementia	Derica
Darlenne	Davyd	Debralee	Delancey	Demeter	Dericia
Darlina	Davyzha	Debs	Delaney	Demetra	Dericka
Darline	Davyzheia	Decca	Delaware	Demetria	Derinda
Darlita	Daw	December	Delcine	Demi	Derine

Derora	Destiny	Dezirae	Dilana	Dmitrovna	Donatella
Derorice	Destry	Deziree	Dilanne	Doanna	Donaver
Derorit	Desyre	Dhana	Dillian	Doanne	Donda
Derrica	Detana	Dhara	Dillon	Dobegneva	Donella
Derring	Detava	Dharma	Dilly	Dobislava	Donelle
Derry	Detta	Dhavala	Dilys	Dobka	Donetta
Derska	Deularla	Dhyana	Dima	Dobra	Donielle
Derval	Deva	Di	Dimaia	Dobrava	Donier
Dervilia	Devaki	Dia	Dimanche	Dobreva	Donisha
Dervla	Devan	Diablo	Dimitra	Dobromila	Donna
Dervorgilla	Devana	Diah	Dimity	Dobroslava	Donna-marie
Derwen	Devaney	Diahann	Dimona	Dobrowest	Donnalee
Derya	Devanie	Diahna	Dimut	Dobryna	Donnalyn
Deryn	Devanna	Diamanda	Dina	Docila	Donnelly
Derzhena	Devany	Diamanta	Dinah	Doda	Donni
Derzhka	Deven	Diamond	Dinara	Dodie	Donnica
Des	Devenny	Diamonique	Dinna	Doe	Donnie
Desa	Devent	Diamontina	Dinora	Doga	Donoma
Desarae	Devera	Dian	Dinorah	Doireann	Donya
Desaree	Devery	Diana	Dion	Dollie	Doon
Desdemona	Devi	Diandra	Diona	Dolly	Doone
Deserae	Devica	Diane	Dione	Dolores	Dora
Deseronto	Devika	Dianna	Dionis	Dolorita	Dorabella
Desha	Devin	Diannah	Dionisa	Domani	Doralia
Desi	Devinee	Dianne	Dionna	Domaslava	Doralie
Desideria	Devka	Diantha	Dionne	Domela	Doralynn
Desir	Devnet	Dianthe	Dionysia	Domele	Dorbeta
Desirae	Devo	Diara	Dionysie	Domenica	Dorcas
Desiraee	Devochka	Diarra	Dior	Domiduca	Dorcey
Desirat	Devochkina	Diarria	Diorbhall	Domina	Dordei
Desire	Devon	Diaz	Dirce	Dominga	Dordie
Desiree	Devona	Dicra	Disa	Domini	Dore
Desirrae	Devondra	Didi	Discovery	Dominica	Doreen
Desirus	Devonee	Didiane	Dita	Dominik	Dorene
Desislava	Devonna	Didina	Ditza	Dominika	Doretta
Desma	Devonne	Dido	Diva	Dominique	Dori
Despa	Devony	Didrika	Diversity	Domino	Doria
Despina	Devora	Diedre	Divina	Domitiane	Dorian
Dessa	Devorah	Diega	Divine	Domitilla	Doriana
Dessirae	Devoria	Diella	Divinity	Domitille	Doriann
Desta	Devorit	Dielle	Divna	Domka	Dorianna
Destanee	Devra	Diem	Divsha	Domna	Dorie
Destina	Devri	Diep	Divshah	Domnika	Dorielle
Destinarea	Devyn	Dierdra	Divya	Domnikiia	Dorika
Destine	Devynn	Dierdre	Diwata	Domnina	Dorinda
Destinee	Dex	Difyr	Dixie	Domona	Dorine
Destiney	Dexter	Digna	Diza	Dona	Doris
Destini	Dextra	Dija	Djuna	Donae	Dorit
Destinie	Deyanira	Dikana	Dmitreeva	Donalda	Dorita
Destinny	Deysi	Dikla	Dmitrieva	Donata	Dorkas

78

Dorma	Drga	Dustee	Earlina	Edie	Efrosini
Doro	Drina	Dusti	Early	Edilburga	Efrossina
Doroata	Drosida	Dustin	Earna	Ediline	Egberta
Dorofeia	Dru	Dustine	Earnestyna	Edina	Egbertina
Dorona	Drue	Dusty	Eartha	Edine	Egbertine
Dorote	Drucilla	Dusya	Earwyn	Edita	Egbertyne
Dorotea	Druella	Duvessa	Earwyna	Edith	Egelina
Doroteia	Drum	Duyen	East	Editta	Egeria
Doroteya	Drury	Dvora	Easter	Edlen	Egidia
Dorothea	Drusilla	Dwi	Easton	Edlyn	Eglantina
Dorothee	Druzhinina	Dwyn	Eathelin	Edmanda	Eglantine
Dorothy	Drysi	Dwynwen	Eathelyn	Edmee	Egle
Dorra	Du	Dyan	Eavan	Edmonda	Egypt
Dorri	Duaa	Dyana	Eban	Edmunda	Eheubryd
Dorrie	Duana	Dyani	Ebba	Edna	Eibhlhin
Dorris	Duayna	Dyann	Ebbony	Ednah	Eibhlin
Dorrit	Dubhain	Dyanna	Ebele	Edolie	Eiddwen
Dorsey	Dubheasa	Dyanne	Eberta	Edra	Eideann
Dorte	Dublin	Dylan	Ebonee	Edraele	Eidel
Dortha	Dubrava	Dylana	Ebonii	Edrea	Eider
Dory	Dubravka	Dylis	Ebonique	Edria	Eifiona
Dosya	Duci	Dyllis	Ebony	Edrice	Eigra
Dot	Dudee	Dymphna	Ebrill	Edris	Eike
Dott	Duena	Dympna	Ebrilla	Eduarda	Eila
Dottie	Duff	Dyna	Ecaeris	Eduardo	Eilat
Dotty	Duffy	Dynah	Ecatarina	Edviga	Eileen
Douce	Duha	Dyre	Ecaterina	Edviva	Eileene
Douglas	Duilya	Dysis	Ecatrinna	Edwardina	Eilena
Dounia	Dukine		Eccentricity	Edwardine	Eilene
Doutzen	Dukinea	**E**	Ece	Edwige	Eilidh
Dove	Duklida		Echo	Edwina	Eilinora
Doveva	Dulce	Eabha	Ecru	Edwinna	Eilionoir
Downeti	Dulcea	Eachna	Eda	Edyta	Eilir
Downett	Dulcia	Eada	Edalene	Edyte	Eilis
Dozene	Dulcibella	Eadan	Edaline	Edyth	Eilise
Dozhene	Dulcie	Eadda	Edan	Edythe	Eilish
Dracen	Dulcina	Eadmund	Edana	Eeva	Eilley
Draginia	Dulcinea	Eadoin	Edda	Eevi	Eilonwy
Dragomira	Dulcinia	Eadwine	Eddith	Efa	Eilwen
Dragoslawa	Dumia	Eagle	Edee	Efdokia	Eily
Dragushla	Dune	Ealasaid	Edeen	Effie	Eimear
Draia	Dunixi	Ealga	Edelburga	Effimia	Einat
Draupnir	Dunne	Eallyrl	Edeline	Effy	Einin
Drea	Dunya	Eara	Edelmira	Efharis	Einya
Dream	Dunyasha	Earhart	Eden	Efimia	Eir
Dreama	Durable	Earie	Edena	Efiopskaia	Eira
Dree	Durriyah	Earla	Edenia	Efrasiia	Eire
Dreena	Dusana	Earleen	Edeva	Efrat	Eireen
Dresden	Duscha	Earlena	Edga	Efrata	Eirene
Drew	Dusha	Earlene	Edge	Efrosenia	Eirian

Eiric	Eldoris	Eliana	Ellylw	Elliza	Elwira
Eirica	Eldreda	Eliane	Eliza	Ellizabeth	Elwyn
Eiriol	Eldrida	Elianna	Elizabella	Ellora	Elwyna
Eirlys	Elea	Elias	Elizabet	Ellowyn	Elya
Eirny	Eleadora	Eliava	Elizabeth	Ellsa	Elyce
Eirwen	Eleana	Elicia	Elizabetta	Ellsie	Elynn
Eirwyn	Eleanor	Elidi	Elizarova	Elly	Elysa
Eiry	Eleanora	Elidia	Elizaveta	Ellyn	Elyse
Eisa	Eleanore	Elie	Elizza	Ellyse	Elysha
Eistir	Electa	Elienor	Elka	Ellysia	Elysia
Eithna	Electra	Elif	Elkana	Elm	Elyssa
Eithne	Eleena	Eligia	Elke	Elma	Elysse
Eivor	Eleftheria	Elikapeka	Ella	Elmina	Elyssia
Eka	Elegance	Elikonida	Ellaina	Elmira	Elyta
Ekanta	Elegia	Elili	Ellaine	Elnora	Elza
Ekat	Elektra	Elin	Ellamae	Elodia	Elzbeta
Ekatarina	Elen	Elina	Ellarian	Elodie	Elzbieta
Ekaterina	Elena	Elinda	Ellasyn	Eloen	Elzhbeta
Ekatrinna	Elenaril	Eline	Ellayne	Eloisa	Elzira
Ekin	Elene	Elinor	Elle	Eloise	Ema
Ekko	Eleni	Elinore	Elleanor	Eloisee	Emalee
Ekundayo	Elenna	Eliora	Elleen	Elon	Eman
Ekzuperiia	Elenora	Eliot	Ellema	Elonka	Emani
Ela	Elenore	Elira	Ellen	Eloquent	Emanita
Elacha	Elenya	Elisa	Ellena	Elora	Emanuela
Elaina	Eleonara	Elisabet	Ellene	Elowen	Emanuele
Elaine	Eleonora	Elisabeth	Elleni	Elpida	Ember
Elainna	Eleonore	Elisabetta	Ellenor	Elrica	Emberlei
Elam	Eleora	Elisae	Elleree	Els	Emberly
Elan	Eleri	Elisamarie	Ellery	Elsa	Emberlyn
Elana	Eleta	Elisava	Ellesse	Elsbeth	Emberlynn
Elanah	Eletha	Elisavet	Ellette	Else	Embeth
Elanalue	Elethea	Elisaveta	Elli	Elsie	Embla
Elandra	Elethia	Elise	Ellia	Elske	Embry
Elani	Eletta	Elish	Elliana	Elspeth	Emelda
Elanie	Elettra	Elisha	Elliann	Elu	Emele
Elanil	Eleuthera	Elisheba	Ellianna	Elula	Emelia
Elanna	Eleutheria	Elisheva	Ellice	Eluned	Emelie
Elara	Eleven	Elishia	Ellie	Elva	Emelin
Elasha	Elexis	Elisia	Ellina	Elvena	Emelina
Elata	Elfreda	Eliska	Ellington	Elvera	Emeline
Elaxi	Elfrida	Elissa	Ellinor	Elvi	Emely
Elayna	Elfrieda	Elissabeth	Elliot	Elvia	Emelyn
Elba	Elga	Elisse	Elliott	Elvie	Emeny
Elberta	Elgielyn	Elissha	Ellis	Elvina	Emer
Elberte	Elgiva	Elita	Ellisa	Elvinia	Emera
Elbertina	Eli	Elitia	Ellise	Elvira	Emerald
Elbertyna	Elia	Elixyvett	Ellisha	Elvis	Emeraude
Elda	Eliada	Elixyvette	Ellison	Elvita	Emerence
Eldora	Eliaksha	Eliya	Ellissa	Elvyne	Emerie

Emerson	Emunah	Epifania	Ermolina	Estefanny	Eugenie
Emersyn	Ena	Epikhariia	Erna	Estefany	Eula
Emery	Enat	Epiphany	Ernesta	Esteffany	Eulala
Emese	Encarna	Epistima	Ernestina	Estela	Eulalia
Emesta	Encarnaci	Epona	Ernestine	Estelita	Eulalie
Emi	Encarnacion	Eponine	Eroica	Estella	Euleta
Emiko	Enchantra	Eppie	Erotiida	Estelle	Euna
Emilee	Enda	Era	Errica	Estephanie	Eunice
Emileigh	Endeavor	Erasto	Errigal	Ester	Euphemia
Emiley	Endellion	Ercilia	Errika	Esteva	Euphrates
Emili	Endora	Erdudvyl	Errin	Esther	Euphrosyne
Emilia	Energy	Erela	Erryn	Estienne	Euprakseia
Emiliana	Eneuawg	Erelah	Erscilia	Eston	Eupraksiia
Emilie	Enfys	Erendira	Ersilia	Estralita	Eurfron
Emiliee	Engelbertha	Erendiria	Erskina	Estrela	Euridice
Emiliya	Engelbertina	Erene	Ertugana	Estrella	Eurneid
Emillia	Engelbertine	Eres	Erwina	Estrellita	Euroa
Emillie	Engla	Eretiia	Erwyna	Estrid	EurolwVn
Emilly	England	Erga	Eryn	Esyae	Euron
Emily	Engleberta	Eri	Erynn	Esyllt	Euronwy
Emina	Engracia	Erica	Erzsebet	Eszter	Eurwen
Emira	Enid	Ericca	Esadowa	Eta	Eurydice
Emke	Eniko	Ericka	Esarosa	Etain	Eusebia
Emlen	Eniola	Eridian	Eshana	Etana	Eustace
Emlyn	Enit	Erie	Eshe	Etel	Eustacia
Emma	Enite	Erika	Eshenesra	Etelburga	Euzebia
Emmalee	Enjoli	Erikka	Esineeva	Etenia	Eva
Emmalia	Enna	Eriko	Eskama	Eternity	Eva Marie
Emmaline	Ennafa	Erimentha	Eskame	Ethel	Eva-Yolanda
Emmalyn	Ennis	Erin	Esma	Ethelberta	Evacska
Emmalynn	Enola	Erina	Esme	Ethelda	Evadine
Emmanuella	Enora	Eris	Esmeralda	Etheldreda	Evadne
Emmanuelle	Enrhydreg	Erisha	Esmeraude	Ethelinda	Evaline
Emmanulle	Enrica	Erith	Esmerelda	Ethelred	Evalisse
Emmarald	Enrichetta	Eritha	Esmerie	Ethereal	Evalyn
Emme	Enrika	Erizelda	Esperanza	Ethical	Evalyse
Emmeline	Enriqua	Erla	Espn	Ethna	Evan
Emmet	Enriqueta	Erlat	Essaerae	Ethne	Evana
Emmett	Enterprise	Erlene	Essence	Etilka	Evangelia
Emmi	Entropy	Erlina	Essery	Etney	Evangelina
Emmilia	Eny	Erlinda	Essi	Etoile	Evangeline
Emmilie	Enya	Erline	Essie	Etsuko	Evania
Emmily	Enye	Erling	Esta	Etta	Evanna
Emmly	Enyo	Erma	Estacia	Etty	Evanova
Emmy	Enza	Ermelinde	Este	Etude	Evans
Emmylou	Eolande	Ermengard	Estebana	Euafina	Evanthe
Emory	Eos	Ermengarde	Estee	Eudocia	Evdokeia
Empress	Eowyn	Ermina	Estefana	Eudora	Evdokia
Emsley	Epestemiia	Ermine	Estefani	Eufemia	Evdokiia
Emuna	Ephiphany	Ermintrude	Estefania	Eugenia	Evdokiya

Evdokseia	Evline	Fahari	Farina	Fedella	Fennel
Evdoksiia	Evon	Fahima	Farley	Fedelma	Fennella
Eve	Evonna	Faida	Farrah	Federica	Fenya
Eve Marie	Evonne	Faiga	Farran	Fedia	Feodora
Evea	Evonnia	Faina	Farrell	Fedka	Feodosia
Evee	Evony	Fainche	Farren	Fedkina	Feodosiia
Eveleen	Evpraksi	Faine	Farryn	Fedora	Feoduliia
Evelia	Evpraksiia	Fairen	Farsiris	Fedoritsa	Feofana
Evelien	Evrose	Fairfax	Farva	Fedorka	Feoklita
Evelin	Evrosena	Fairlee	Farzaneh	Fedorova	Feoktista
Evelina	Evseevskaia	Fairly	Fate	Fedosia	Feona
Eveline	Evsegniia	Fairuza	Fathia	Fedosiia	Feonilla
Evelinn	Evseveia	Fairyn	Fathiyya	Fedosya	Feopimta
Evella	Evseviia	Faith	Fatianova	Fedotia	Feopista
Evellyn	Evstoliia	Faithe	Fatima	Fedotiia	Feopistiia
Evelyn	Evtropiia	Faizah	Fatimah	Fedya	Feozva
Evelyne	Evva	Fala	Fatin	Fee	Ferebee
Evelynn	Evvie	Falala	Fatma	Feechi	Ferelith
Evening	Evynne	Falan	Faun	Feenat	Fereshteh
Evensong	Ewa	Falcon	Fauna	Feia	Ferfufiia
Ever	Ewelina	Faline	Faunalyn	Feiniia	Fergie
Evera	Exaltacion	Fallon	Faunia	Fekla	Fermina
Everest	Exodus	Fallyn	Faunus	Feklitsa	Fern
Everett	Experience	Falon	Fausta	Fela	Fernanda
Everil	Explorer	Famke	Faustina	Felberta	Fernande
Everleigh	Eydie	Fana	Faustine	Felda	Fernley
Everly	Eyota	Fanaila	Fauve	Felecia	Ferrari
Everlyn	Eyre	Fanchon	Favor	Felice	Ferufa
Everlyse	Eyslk	Fanchone	Favsta	Felicia	Feryal
Evert	Ezmeralda	Fancy	Fawn	Felician	Fesalonikiia
Every	Ezra	Fanetta	Fawnia	Felicidad	Fetenia
Evette	Ezri	Fanette	Fawzia	Felicienne	Fetinia
Evfaliia	Ezria	Fani	Fay	Felicita	Fetiniia
Evfrasiia	Eztli	Fania	Fayanna	Felicitas	Fevronia
Evfroseniia		Fanni	Faydell	Felicity	Fews
Evfrosinya	**F**	Fannia	Faye	Feline	Fey
Evgenia		Fannie	Fayette	Felisa	Feya
Evgeniia	Fabia	Fanny	Fayina	Felisha	Ffanci
Evgeniya	Fabiana	Fantasia	Faylinn	Felixa	Ffion
Evgenya	Fabianna	Fantina	Fayme	Felka	Fflur
Evginia	Fabianne	Fantine	Fayola	Fellicia	Ffraid
Evguenia	Fabienne	Fanya	Fayre	Femi	Fhaertala
Evia	Fabiola	Faqueza	Fayruz	Feminista	Fia
Evian	Fable	Farah	Fayth	Femke	Fiachina
Eviana	Fabrizia	Farasha	Faythe	Fenella	Fiachra
Evie	Fabunni	Fareeda	Fealty	Feng	Fiala
Evike	Fadia	Faren	Fearchara	Fenia	Fiammetta
Evina	Fadila	Farica	Fearcharia	Fenmore	Fiana
Evita	Fae	Farida	Feather	Fenna	Fianait
Evlin	Faelyn	Farin	February	Fenne	Fianna

82

Fiby	Fionna	Floriane	Frances	Friederike	Gafnit
Fidda	Fionnghuala	Florida	Francesca	Frigg	Gaho
Fidelia	Fionnuala	Florie	Francess	Frikka	Gaia
Fidelina	Fionnula	Florinda	Francessca	Fritha	Gaiana
Fideline	Fiora	Florinia	Franchesca	Fritzi	Gaianiia
Fidelity	Fiorella	Floris	Francille	Fritzie	Gail
Fidella	Fiorenza	Florissa	Francina	Frolova	Gailine
Fidelma	Fira	Florita	Francine	Frosiniia	Gaille
Fiducia	Firenze	Floriza	Francique	Frost	Gainell
Fieryat	Firoza	Florrie	Francisca	Frostine	Gaira
Fiesta	Firth	Flory	Franciszka	Fructuosa	Gajijens
Fife	Firtha	Flossie	Francoise	Fruma	Gal
Fifer	Fiva	Flower	Françoise	Fuchsia	Gala
Fifi	Fiveia	Floy	Franisbel	Fuensanta	Galatea
Fifine	Fizza	Floyce	Franka	Fukayna	Galatee
Fifna	Fjola	Flynn	Franki	Fulgencia	Galatia
Fifne	Fjord	Flyta	Frankie	Fulvia	Galaxy
Fig	Flaca	Foimina	Frankie-jean	Fumiko	Gale
Filaurel	Flair	Fokina	Frannie	Future	Galen
Filauria	Flame	Fola	Franny	Fyfa	Galena
Fildaerae	Flaminia	Folami	Franziska	Fynballa	Galenia
Filia	Flana	Folasade	Frayda	Fyodora	Galenka
Filicia	Flanders	Fomina	Fraydel		Gali
Filikitata	Flann	Fonda	Freda	**G**	Galia
Filipa	Flanna	Fone	Freddi		Galiana
Filipina	Flannerry	Fontanne	Freddie	Gabbriel	Galice
Filippa	Flannery	Forba	Freddy	Gabbriella	Galiena
Filippiia	Flash	Forbia	Fredella	Gabby	Galila
Filis	Flavia	Forest	Frederica	Gabi	Galilah
Filitsata	Flavie	Forever	Frederique	Gable	Galilahi
Filofei	Flede	Forsythia	Fredrica	Gabrianna	Galilaia
Filofinaia	Fleta	Fortney	Fredricka	Gabrie	Galilea
Filomena	Fleur	Fortuna	Fredrika	Gabriela	Galilee
Filonilla	Fleurette	Fortunata	Free	Gabriele	Galilhai
Fimochka	Flick	Fortune	Freedom	Gabriella	Galina
Fina	Flo	Fortuo	Freesia	Gabrielle	Galine
Finch	Floella	Fotina	Freida	Gabrina	Galit
Fineena	Flor	Fotiniia	Freira	Gaby	Galla
Finella	Flora	Fountain	Freja	Gada	Gallia
Fini	Floramaria	Fovro	French	Gadar	Galochka
Finlay	Flordeperia	Fovroneia	Frenchie	Gadina	Galway
Finley	Florence	Foxie	Frenchy	Gaea	Galya
Finn	Florencia	Foxy	Frescura	Gael	Galyna
Finna	Florentina	Foy	Freya	Gaelira	Gamana
Finnea	Florenza	Fran	Frida	Gaenor	Gambhira
Finnegan	Floressa	Franca	Frideborg	Gaerradh	Gambhiri
Finola	Floretta	Franccesca	Frideswide	Gaerwen	Gamila
Finula	Flori	France	Frieda	Gaetana	Gamma
Fiona	Floria	Francena	Friedegarde	Gaetane	Gana
Fionn	Floriana	Francene	Friedelinde	Gafna	Gananiia

83

Gandaza	Gaye	Geneva	Gerlinde	Gili	Glynna
Ganesa	Gayatri	Genevalisse	Germain	Gilia	Giza
Ganesha	Gayelette	Geneve	Germaine	Gilit	Gizeh
Ganet	Gayla	Genevie	Germana	Gillian	Gizela
Ganice	Gayle	Genevieve	Gerry	Gimbya	Gizheurann
Ganit	Gaylee	Genevra	Gersemi	Gin	Gizi
Ganna	Gaylia	Genevre	Gertrud	Gina	Gizla
Gannet	Gayna	Genica	Gertruda	Ginata	Gjertrud
Ganya	Gaynell	Genisa	Gertrude	Ginechka	Glade
Gaphna	Gaynor	Genisia	Gertrudes	Ginerva	Gladis
Gara	Gayora	Genista	Gertrudia	Ginette	Gladys
Garabina	Gazella	Genivee	Gertrudis	Ginevra	Glafira
Garabine	Gazelle	Genka	Gertrut	Ginger	Glain
Garaitz	Gazit	Genna	Gerusha	Ginna	Glan
Garan	Geavonna	Gennesis	Gervaise	Ginnette	Glasgow
Garbina	Gechina	Gennevieve	Gesine	Ginnie	Glasha
Garbine	Geela	Gennifer	Gethsemane	Ginnifer	Glaucia
Garbo	Geena	Genoa	Geulah	Ginny	Glaw
Garcelle	Geertruida	Genova	Geva	Gioconda	Glebovicha
Garcia	Gefen	Genoveva	Gevira	Gioia	Gleda
Garden	Gefion	Gentry	Gezana	Giolla	Glenda
Gardener	Gefjun	Geona	Ghada	Giordana	Glenn
Gardenia	Geila	Geonna	Ghadir	Giorgianna	Glenna
Gardner	Gelasia	Georgeann	Ghaliya	Giovana	Glennda
Gari	Gelilah	Georgeanna	Ghilanna	Giovanna	Glennis
Garia	Gella	Georgeanne	Ghislaine	Gisa	Glenys
Garima	Gelsey	Georgene	Ghita	Gisbelle	Glikeriia
Garin	Gelsomina	Georgette	Gia	Gisel	Glikeriya
Garland	Gem	Georgia	Giacinta	Gisela	Glimmer
Garnet	Gema	Georgiana	Giada	Gisele	Glinda
Garsteaode	Gemala	Georgianna	Giana	Gisella	Gliona
Gary	Gemelle	Georgianne	Gianara	Giselle	Glison
Garyn	Gemi	Georgie	Gianetta	Gish	Glora
Gasha	Gemini	Georgieva	Gianina	Gisli	Gloria
Gaspara	Gemma	Georgina	Gianna	Gisselle	Gloriann
Gatlin	Gemstarzah	Georgine	Giannina	Gita	Glorianne
Gattaca	Gen	Georgitte	Giavanna	Gitana	Glormarie
Gauge	Gena	Geovana	Gidget	Gitel	Glory
Gaura	Gene	Geovany	Gidja	Githa	Gluckel
Gauri	Genee	Geraldene	Gift	Gitta	Glukeriia
Gavenia	Geneen	Geraldine	Gigi	Gittel	Glukheria
Gavi	Genera	Geralyn	Gil	Giuditta	Glyn
Gavina	Generosa	Geranium	Gila	Giulia	Glynae
Gavra	Generosity	Gerarda	Gilah	Giuliana	Glynda
Gavriela	Genesee	Gerardine	Gilal	Giurgevaia	Glynis
Gavriella	Genesis	Gerd	Gilala	Giuseppina	Glynn
Gavrila	Genesiss	Gerda	Gilana	Giustina	Glynnii
Gavrilla	Genessa	Gerdie	Gilbarta	Giustinia	Glynnis
Gavyn	Genessis	Geri	Gilberte	Giverny	Gnishilda
Gay	Genet	Gerianne	Gilda	Glyn	Gobinet

Gobnait	Gracelyn	Grietje	Gunesh	Gwenore	Hafsah
Gobnat	Gracelynn	Grifina	Gunhilda	Gwenyth	Hafwen
Godava	Gracelynne	Grigoreva	Gunhilde	Gweyr	Hagar
Goddess	Gracen	Grigorevna	Gunilla	Gwladus	Haide
Godeleine	Gracia	Grigorieva	Gunna	Gwladys	Haidee
Godeleva	Gracie	Grisel	Gunnef	Gwylan	Haile
Godelieve	Graciee	Griselda	Gunnel	Gwyn	Hailee
Godfreya	Graciela	Griselde	Gunnhild	Gwyndolen	Haileigh
Godgifu	Gracyn	Griseldis	Gunnhilde	Gwyndolin	Hailey
Godiva	Grady	Griselle	Guri	Gwyndolyn	Haili
Goewin	Graina	Grishilde	Gurice	Gwynedd	Hailie
Golda	Grainne	Grizel	Gurit	Gwyneira	Hailley
Golden	Gráinne	Grizela	Gus	Gwyneth	Hailly
Goldie	Granada	Grizelda	Gussie	Gwynith	Haily
Goldine	Grande	Grove	Gust	Gwynn	Hajar
Golds	Grania	Groza	Gusta	Gwynne	Hajra
Goldy	Granthana	Gruba	Gustava	Gwynnestri	Hakan
Goleuddydd	Gratia	Grunya	Gustel	Gwynneth	Hakidonmuya
Golindukha	Gratiana	Grusha	Gustey	Gyda	Hala
Golnaz	Gravity	Grushilda	Gusty	Gyldan	Halaema
Goltiaeva	Gravriia	Gryphon	Guthrie	Gylledha	Halah
Golubitsa	Gray	Gryta	Gutka	Gypsy	Halanaestra
Gopi	Grazia	Guadalupe	Gwaeddan	Gzifa	Halcyon
Gorasgwrn	Graziana	Guadelupe	Gwanwyn		Halcyone
Gorawen	Graziella	Guanina	Gwawr	**H**	Haldana
Gordana	Grazina	Gubnat	Gwen		Haldis
Gordania	Grazinia	Gucci	Gwenabwy	Habiba	Haldisa
Gordislava	Grazyna	Gudrid	Gwenaelle	Habibah	Haleigh
Gorislava	Grear	Gudrun	Gwenda	Hacathra	Halen
Gormghlaith	Green	Guendolina	Gwendelyn	Hachi	Halette
Gormley	Greenlee	Guenevere	Gwendi	Hada	Haley
Gormly	Greenleigh	Guernsey	Gwendolen	Hadar	Halfrid
Gorshedna	Greer	Guevara	Gwendoline	Hadara	Halfrida
Gossamer	Greeta	Guida	Gwendoloena	Hadarah	Hali
Gostena	Gregoria	Guiditta	Gwendolyn	Hadas	Halia
Gostenia	Greige	Guiliaine	Gwendolynn	Hadasa	Halie
Gostiata	Grekina	Guilie	Gwener	Hadasah	Halima
Gostimira	Grekinia	Guillelmina	Gweneth	Hadassah	Halimah
Gota	Grekyna	Guillermina	Gwenevere	Haddie	Halimeda
Gote	Greta	Guinevere	Gwenfair	Hadeya	Halina
Gotilda	Gretal	Guiseppina	Gwenhwyvar	Hadia	Hallam
Goulislava	Gretchen	Guitain	Gwenifer	Hadiya	Halldora
Govdela	Gretchine	Guitar	Gwenith	Hadlee	Halle
Goya	Grete	Gul	Gwenledyr	Hadleigh	Halleigh
Grace	Gretel	Guliana	Gwenllian	Hadley	Halleli
Graceann	Gretta	Gulielma	Gwenn	Hadrea	Halley
Graceanne	Grey	Gull	Gwenna	Hadria	Halli
Gracee	Grid	Gulzar	GwennAlarch	Haeley	Hallie
Graceland	Grier	Gunda	Gwennan	Haf	Halo
Gracella	Griet	Gundruna	Gwenno	Hafsa	Halona

Halsey	Harleen	Hawaii	Helga	Hestia	Hita
Halyn	Harleigh	Haya	Helge	Hetal	Hitee
Halyna	Harlem	Haydée	Helia	Hetta	Hitomi
Hamako	Harlene	Hayden	Helisent	Hettie	Hjördis
Hamalitia	Harlequin	Hayfa	Helki	Hetty	Hjørdis
Hamida	Harley	Hayle	Hellen	Heulwen	Hodawa
Hamilton	Harleyann	Haylea	Hellena	Heulwens	Hodaya
Hamo	Harli	Haylee	Heloise	Hialeah	Hokaratcha
Hana	Harlie	Hayleigh	Helsa	Hiba	Hokona
Hanaa	Harlow	Hayley	Hema	Hibah	Hoku
Hanae	Harmonia	Hayli	Hemera	Hibernia	Holda
Hanah	Harmonie	Haylie	Hendrika	Hibiscus	Holiday
Hanako	Harmony	Hayliee	Hendrina	Hide	Hollace
Hang	Harolyn	Hayllie	Henia	Hidi	Holland
Hanh	Harper	Hazel	Henie	Hien	Hollee
Hani	Harriet	Hazelle	Heniuta	Hija	Holleen
Hania	Harriett	Hazina	Henka	Hikari	Holley
Hanifa	Harrietta	Hazzel	Henley	Hikaru	Holli
Hanita	Harriette	Hea	Henna	Hikmat	Hollie
Hanna	Harsha	Heather	Hennessy	Hila	Hollis
Hannah	Hartley	Heaven	Hennie	Hilaire	Holly
Hannalee	Harue	Heavenly	Henoheno	Hilaria	Hollyann
Hannan	Haruhi	Heba	Henrietta	Hilary	Hollyn
Hanne	Haruka	Hebe	Henriette	Hilda	Holone
Hannela	Haruko	Hecuba	Henrika	Hilde	Honbria
Hannele	Harum	Hedda	Henrike	Hildegard	Honesty
Hannelore	Harumi	Hedia	Henuita	Hildegarde	Honey
Hanny	Haruna	Hedva	Henuite	Hildemar	Hong
Hanrietta	Harva	Hedvige	Henya	Hildireth	Honna
Hanriette	Hasana	Hedwig	Hephzibah	Hildreth	Honoka
Hansika	Hasina	Hedy	Hepsiba	Hillary	Honor
Hansine	Hasna	Hedya	Hepzibah	Hilliard	Honora
Hanzila	Hateya	Hege	Hepzibeth	Hilma	Honorata
Hao	Hathor	Hehewuti	Heqet	Himalaya	Honore
Happy	Hatshepsut	Heide	Hera	Himani	Honoria
Haqikah	Hatsu	Heidi	Heriberto	Himawari	Honorina
Hara	Hatsy	Heidrun	Hermandina	Hina	Honorine
Haracha	Hattie	Heidy	Hermia	Hinata	Honour
Haralda	Hatty	Heike	Herminia	Hinda	Honovi
Haramara	Haukea	Hekuba	Hermione	Hindel	Honza
Haranu	Hausis	Heladia	Hermip	Hinezka	Hoowanneka
Harbor	Hausisse	Helaine	Hermosa	Hinica	Hop
Harding	Hava	Helartha	Hero	Hinto	Hope
Harela	Havana	Heleen	Herodias	Hiolair	Hopeton
Hariata	Haven	Heleena	Hersilia	Hippolyta	Hora
Harika	Havilah	Helen	Hertha	Hippolyte	Horatia
Haripriya	Havily	Helena	Hesper	Hiraani	Horina
Harlan	Haviva	Helene	Hesperia	Hiroko	Horizon
Harlean	Havva	Helenka	Hessa	Hisano	Hortense
Harlee	Hawa	Helenna	Hester	Hisolda	Hortensia

Hortenspa	Iakova	Idella	Ilayda	Imani	Inga
Hosa	Iakovleva	Idelle	Ilde	Imanii	Ingaborg
Hosanna	Iakovlevskaia	Iden	Ildiko	Imanni	Ingalill
Hosannah	Iakun	Idetta	Ildilyntra	Imara	Inge
Hosche	Iakunova	Idina	Ildri	Imee	Ingeborg
Hoshi	Iakunovaia	Idit	Ileana	Imelda	Ingegard
Hoshiko	Ialantha	Idla	Ilena	Imena	Ingenue
Hostena	Ianevaia	Idola	Ilene	Imizael	Inger
Hourig	Ianisha	Idona	Ilesha	Imke	Inghean
Hova	Ianishe	Idonia	Ilham	Immaculada	Inghinn
Howard	Ianka	Idony	Ilia	Immani	Ingri
Howea	Ianna	Idra	Iliana	Immianthe	Ingrid
Hrefna	Iantha	Idris	Ilianna	Immogene	Ingvil
Hristina	Ianthe	Iduia	Ilima	Immy	Ingvild
Hruoza	Iara	Idun	Ilina	Imogen	Ingvill
Huali	Iarche	Iduna	Ilisa	Imogene	Iniabi
Huberta	Iarena	Ieesha	Ilise	Imogenia	Iniga
Huda	Iarina	Iekeliene	Ilisha	Imperia	Inika
Hudson	Iarogned	Iekika	Ilissa	Imra	Iniko
Hue	Iaroia	Ieliaia	Ilithya	Imryll	Inis
Huela	Iarokhna	Ierne	Iliya	Ina	Inka
Huette	Iaroslava	Iev	Ilka	Inali	Inkena
Hugette	Iarshek	Ievlia	Ilkay	Inara	Inmaculada
Huguetta	Iasynia	Ifama	Illeana	Inari	Inna
Huguette	Iban	Ife	Illiana	Inaya	Innes
Hulda	Ibby	Ifrosenia	Illianna	Inbal	Innis
Humaira	Iberia	Ignacia	Illinois	Inbar	Ino
Humility	Ibernia	Ignateva	Illumination	Inca	Inoa
Humita	Ibis	Ignatevskaia	Illuminée	Inci	Inocencia
Humla	Ibolya	Igoshkova	Illusion	Indah	Inoceneia
Hummer	Ibtesam	Igraine	Ilma	Indeg	Inocenta
Humvee	Ica	Iha	Ilmadia	Independence	Inoke
Hunter	Icelyn	Ihuicatl	Ilona	Indi	Inola
Huong	Ichigo	Iia	Ilsa	India	Inspiration
Huquethae	Ichtaca	Iida	Ilse	Indiana	Insula
Hurit	Ickett	Ijlal	Ilsevel	Indianna	Intan
Hurricane	Icnoyotl	Ikaia	Iluminada	Indie	Integra
Huyana	Ida	Ikea	Ily	Indigo	Integrity
Huyen	Idabelle	Ikeshia	Ilva	Indira	Inu
Hyacinth	Idalah	Ikia	Ilyrana	Indiya	Io
Hyancinthe	Idalee	Ikram	Ilys	Indra	Ioanna
Hycis	Idalia	Ikuyo	Ilyssa	Indrajit	Ioelena
Hye	Idalina	Ila	Ilythyrra	Indrani	Ioke
Hypatia	Idalis	Ilana	Ima	Indre	Iokina
Hyria	Idalyz	Ilandere	Imaani	Indu	Iola
	Idana	Ilane	Imagine	Indy	Iolana
I	Idania	Ilanit	Imaging	Ines	Iolani
	Ide	Ilar	Imajica	Inessa	Iolanthe
Iadviga	Ideashia	Ilaria	Imala	Inez	Iona
Iaera	Ideh	Ilariia	Iman	Infinity	Ionanna

Ione	Isaabella	Isolda	Ivey	Jacinda	Jaetyn
Ionia	Isabeau	Isolde	Ivi	Jacinta	Jaffa
Ionna	Isabel	Isondo	Ivie	Jacinth	Jafit
Iorwen	Isabela	Isqesis	Ivonne	Jacintha	Jafita
Iosifova	Isabell	Isra	Ivory	Jacinthe	Jaganmata
Ioulia	Isabella	Israela	Ivria	Jackeline	Jagienka
Iovilla	Isabelle	Issabel	Ivy	Jackie	Jahdahdieh
Iowa	Isabelline	Issabela	Iwalani	Jacklynn	Jahzara
Iphigenia	Isabetta	Issabell	Iwatoke	Jackopa	Jaicee
Iphigenie	Isabis	Issabella	Iwona	Jaclyn	Jaida
Ipo	Isadora	Issis	Ixtli	Jaclynn	Jaide
Ira	Isadorer	Istas	Iyabo	Jacoba	Jaiden
Iraia	Isak	Ita	Iyana	Jacobean	Jaidyn
Iraida	Isakova	Itala	Iyanna	Jacobien	Jailene
Iran	Isaline	Italia	Iyeshia	Jacobina	Jailyn
Iran-dokht	Isandro	Ithaca	Izabella	Jacqualine	Jaime
Irania	Isane	Itiireae	Izar	Jacqueleen	Jaimee
Irati	Isannah	Itka	Izara	Jacqueline	Jaimelynn
Iratze	Isanne	Itotia	Izaro	Jacquelinne	Jaimi
Irayna	Isaura	Itsaso	Izarra	Jacquelle	Jaimie
Irca	Iseabal	Ituha	Izarre	Jacquelline	Jaimilynn
Ireene	Iselin	Itxaro	Izazkun	Jacquelyn	Jaimin
Irela	Isha	Itylra	Izdihar	Jacquelyne	Jaimmie
Ireland	Ishana	Itzel	Ize	Jacquelynn	Jain
Irelyn	Ishara	Iudita	Izefia	Jacquelynne	Jaina
Iren	Ishedus	Iúile	Izel	Jacquenetta	Jaine
Irena	Ishi	Iulia	Izett	Jacquenette	Jaione
Irene	Ishik	Iuliana	Iziaslava	Jacquetta	Jaira
Irhaal	Ishiko	Iulianiia	Izmaragd	Jacqui	Jairdan
Iria	Ishtar	Iulianiii	Izso	Jacy	JaJuan
Irie	Isi	Iuliia	Izumi	Jada	Jakarta
Irina	Isibeal	Iulija	Izusa	Jadda	Jakayla
Irinia	Isidora	Iulita	Izzy	Jade	Jakinda
Irinka	Isilfarrel	Iulitta		Jadee	Jakoba
Iris	Isis	Iuniia	**J**	Jaden	Jakobah
Irisa	Isiss	Iurevna		Jadine	Jala
Irish	Isla	Iustina	Jaada	Jadira	Jalajaa
Irit	Islay	Iva	Jaade	Jadon	Jaleesa
Irka	Isle	Ivah	Jaana	Jadwiga	Jaleh
Irma	Isleen	Ivana	Jaanna	Jadwige	Jalen
Irmina	Islene	Ivane	Jaantje	Jady	Jalena
Irmine	Isley	Ivanka	Jabre	Jadyn	Jalene
Irodia	Ismaela	Ivanna	Jacalyn	Jadzia	Jalessa
Irodiia	Ismagrad	Ivanova	Jacaranda	Jae	Jalia
Irsia	Ismay	Ivanovskaia	Jace	Jaeda	Jalie
Irune	Ismene	Ivara	Jacee	Jael	Jalila
Irus	Isobail	Ivelisse	Jacelyn	Jaela	Jalisa
Irvette	Isobel	Ives	Jacenia	Jaelyn	Jaliyah
Iryna	Isobell	Iveska	Jacey	Jaelynn	Jalyn
Isa	Isoke	Ivette	Jaci	Jaen	Jalynn

88

Jam	Janecia	Jans	Jathbiyya	Jazmyn	Jemima
Jamaica	Janecska	Jansje	Jaunel	Jazmyne	Jemimah
Jamala	Janee	January	Jaunie	Jaznae	Jemina
Jamari	Janeeva	Janus	Java	Jazz	Jemini
Jame	Janell	Janvier	Javier	Jazzelle	Jemma
Jamee	Janella	Jany	Javiera	Jazziell	Jemsa
Jameela	Janelle	Janya	Jawahir	Jazzlyn	Jen
Jameelah	Janese	Jaquelin	Jawdat	Jazzlynn	Jena
Jamese	Janessa	Jaquelina	Jax	Jazzmine	Jenae
Jamesina	Janet	Jaqueline	Jaxine	Jazzmyn	Jenalyn
Jameson	Janeth	Jaquelinee	Jay	Jazzy	Jenalynn
Jamey	Janett	Jaquelinne	Jaya	Jean	Jenara
Jami	Janetta	Jaquelline	Jayana	Jeana	Jenarae
Jamia	Janette	Jaquenetta	Jayane	Jeanay	Jenavieve
Jamie	Janey	Jaquenette	Jayanti	Jeane	Jenay
Jamiee	Jani	Jaquetta	Jayashri	Jeanee	Jenaya
Jamielee	Jania	Jara	Jaycee	Jeanelle	Jenda
Jamii	Janiah	Jarah	Jaycie	Jeanetta	Jendayi
Jamila	Janica	Jardena	Jayda	Jeanette	Jenee
Jamilah	Janice	Jardina	Jayde	Jeanice	Jeneil
Jamilee	Janicia	Jaren	Jayden	Jeanie	Jenelle
Jamilia	Janie	Jarena	Jaye	Jeanina	Jenessa
Jamilla	Janiece	Jarene	Jayla	Jeanine	Jeneth
Jamillah	Janika	Jariah	Jaylaa	Jeaninne	Jenetta
Jamille	Janina	Jarica	Jaylah	Jeann	Jenette
Jamilyn	Janine	Jarita	Jaylee	Jeanna	Jeneva
Jamilynn	Janinne	Jarohna	Jayleen	Jeanne	Jeneve
Jamirah	Janis	Jarrell	Jayleene	Jeannette	Jenevieve
Jamison	Janisa	Jasee	Jaylene	Jeannie	Jenibelle
Jamiya	Janise	Jasia	Jaylenne	Jeannine	Jenica
Jammi	Janita	Jasiri	Jayliah	Jeardra	Jenielle
Jamuna	Janiya	Jasleen	Jaylin	Jearl	Jenifer
Jamya	Janiyah	Jaslene	Jaylyn	Jeaselle	Jeniffer
Jan	Janka	Jaslynn	Jaylynn	Jecolia	Jenifry
Jana	Janli	Jasmeen	Jayme	Jedi	Jenilee
Janaa	Janna	Jasmijn	Jaymee	Jedida	Jenina
Janae	Jannae	Jasmin	Jaymes	Jeena	Jenine
Janaee	Jannah	Jasmine	Jaymi	Jeenifer	Jenis
Janah	Jannalee	Jasminn	Jaymie	Jehane	Jenise
Janai	Janne	Jasminne	Jayna	Jekaterina	Jenita
Janais	Janneke	Jasmyn	Jayne	Jela	Jenna
Janalee	Jannet	Jasmyne	Jaynee	Jelena	Jennabel
Janalyn	Janneth	Jasmynne	Jayni	Jelina	Jennah
Janan	Jannett	Jasna	Jaynie	Jelissa	Jennalee
Janaya	Jannice	Jasone	Jaz	Jelizaveta	Jennalyn
Janaye	Jannie	Jasoslava	Jazlyn	Jellia	Jennasee
Janceena	Jannina	Japser	Jazlynn	Jelsa	Jennavieve
Jancis	Jannine	Jassmin	Jazmin	Jem	Jennaya
Jane	Janny	Jassmine	Jazmine	Jemarie	Jennelle
Janeane	Janoah	Jastra	Jazminne	Jemila	Jennessa

Jennet	Jesimae	Jin	Joeanne	Jomayra	Josephina
Jenneva	Jeslyn	Jina	Joed	Jonalyn	Josephine
Jenni	Jess	Jinan	Joeliyn	Jonatha	Josetta
Jennica	Jessa	Jineen	Joell	jonatha	Josette
Jennie	Jessamina	Jinelle	Joella	Jonati	Joshlynn
Jennifer	Jessamine	Jinendra	Joelle	Jonay	Josie
Jenniferr	Jessamy	Jingjing	Joellen	Jone	Josilyn
Jenniffer	Jessamyn	Jinja	Joelliana	Jonell	Joslin
Jennine	Jesse	Jinni	Joelliane	Jonet	Joslyn
Jennis	Jessenia	Jinny	Joely	Jonetta	Joslynn
Jennison	Jessia	Jinx	Joey	Joni	Joss
Jennlika	Jessica	Jioni	Johana	Jonila	Josselyn
Jennnifer	Jessie	Jira	Johanna	Jonina	Josslyn
Jenny	Jestina	Jiselle	Johannah	Jonna	Josslynn
Jennyfer	Jestine	Jitka	Johari	Jonni	Jostelyn
Jennyl	Jesusa	Jiva	Johnda	Jonnie	Josune
Jensen	Jethra	Jivanta	Johnella	Jonquil	Jourdain
Jensina	Jetje	Jo	Johnelle	Joquil	Journee
Jensine	Jetta	Joakima	Johnetta	Jora	Journey
Jenski	Jette	Joan	Johnna	Jorah	Jovana
Jentry	Jeune	Joana	Johnnie	Jorcina	Jovanna
Jenue	Jevdokija	Joanie	Johyna	Jord	Jovany
Jeorjia	Jeven	Joanka	Joi	Jordan	Jovelyn
Jeovana	Jewel	Joann	Joia	Jordana	Jovena
Jeovanna	Jewell	Joanna	Joie	Jordane	Jovia
Jera	Jezebel	Joanne	Jojo	Jordanna	Jovianne
Jeraldine	Jezel	Joannie	Joka	Jordanne	Jovie
Jeralyn	Jezreel	Joaquina	Joke	Jordence	Jovienne
Jerelyn	Jhanandra	Joaquine	Jokina	Jordyn	Jovina
Jeremia	Jhaumrithe	Jobeth	Jokine	Jordynn	Jovita
Jeremine	Jhiilsraa	Jobey	Jola	Jorgina	Joweese
Jeren	Jia	Jobina	Jolan	Jori	Joxepa
Jereni	JiaLi	Joby	Jolanda	Jorie	Joy
Jeri	Jiana	Jocasta	Jolanta	Jorja	Joya
Jerica	Jiang	Jocelin	Jolee	Jorjanna	Joyann
Jericca	Jicarilla	Jocelina	Joleen	Jorryn	Joyanna
Jericho	Jie	Joceline	Joleene	Jorun	Joyanne
Jeriel	Jihan	Jocellyn	Joleigh	Jory	Joyce
Jerilyn	Jiles	Jocelyn	Jolene	Josalind	Joyceanne
Jermaine	Jilian	Jocelyne	Jolette	Josalyn	Joycee
Jerrely	Jill	Jocelynn	Joli	Josalynn	Joycelyn
Jerrica	Jillene	Jocelynne	Jolie	Joscelyn	Joyelle
Jerricca	Jillian	Jochebed	Jolien	Jose	Joylyn
Jerrie	Jilliane	Jocosa	Jolina	Josebe	Jozlyn
Jerry	Jilliann	Joda	Joline	Josee	Jozsa
Jersey	Jillianna	Jodell	Jolisa	Josefa	Juana
Jerusalem	Jilly	Jodelle	Jolivette	Josefina	Juandalynn
Jerusha	Jimena	Jodi	Jollene	Joselyn	Juanetta
Jesara	Jimenna	Jodie	Jolon	Josepha	Juanisha
Jesenia	Jimi	Jody	Jolyane	Josephe	Juanita

Juanitta	Julita	Kabira	Kailla	Kaliska	Kamilia
Juanna	Julitta	Kace	Kailyn	Kalista	Kamilla
Juba	Julitte	Kacee	Kailynn	Kalitina	Kamille
Jubilee	Jullia	Kaceey	Kaimi	Kaliyah	Kamillra
Juci	Julliana	Kacela	Kainda	Kalla	Kamle
Jucika	Jullianna	Kacey	Kaipo	Kallan	Kammi
Juda	Julliet	Kacha	Kaira	Kallee	Kamryn
Judaea	July	Kache	Kairi	Kalleen	Kana
Judah	Jumana	Kachina	Kaitlan	Kalleigh	Kanai
Jude	Jumanah	Kachka	Kaitleen	Kalley	Kanan
Judeana	Jumelle	Kacia	Kaitlin	Kalli	Kanani
Judee	Jumoke	Kacie	Kaitlinn	Kallie	Kanapima
Judeena	Juna	Kacy	Kaitlyn	Kallima	Kanara
Judi	June	Kade	Kaitlynn	Kalliope	Kandace
Judie	Juneau	Kadee	Kaiya	Kallisfeniia	Kandahl
Judit	Junelle	Kadence	Kaiyo	Kallista	Kandaza
Judith	Junette	Kadenza	Kajol	Kalliyan	Kande
Juditha	Juni	Kadi	Kajsa	Kallyn	Kandice
Judy	Junia	Kadida	Kakalina	Kalona	Kandyl
Jui	Juniper	Kadie	Kakawangwa	Kaloni	Kanga
Juin	Junko	Kadience	Kala	Kalonice	Kani
Juji	Juno	Kadija	Kalama	Kaltha	Kaniesa
Juke	Jurnee	Kadisha	Kalani	Kalyan	Kanika
Jule	Justeen	Kadri	Kalanie	Kalyani	Kanisha
Julee	Justeene	Kady	Kalanit	Kalyca	Kanoa
Juleen	Justice	Kaede	Kalare	Kalyn	Kanon
Jules	Justina	Kaela	Kalea	Kama	Kanoni
Julesa	Justine	Kaelin	Kaleen	Kamaile	Kansas
Juli	Justinne	Kaelyn	Kaleena	Kamala	Kanta
Julia	Justise	Kaelynn	Kalei	Kamali	Kanti
Juliaann	Justyne	Kaena	Kaleigh	Kamana	Kanya
Julian	Jutka	Kaethe	Kalena	Kamara	Kaori
Juliana	Jyl	Kaeya	Kalene	Kamari	Kaoru
Juliane	Jyler	Kagami	Kaleria	Kamaria	Kapena
Juliann	Jyll	Kahlilia	Kaleriia	Kamber	Kapetolina
Julianna	Jyllina	Kahlo	Kaley	Kambria	Kapila
Julianne	Jyoti	Kai	Kali	Kamea	Kapono
Julie	Jyotika	Kaia	Kalia	Kameko	Kapri
Julienne	Jyotis	Kaialani	Kalida	Kamela	Kaptelina
Juliet		Kaida	Kalie	Kamelia	Kara
Julieta	**K**	Kaidence	Kalifa	Kamella	Karah
Juliett		Kaige	Kalii	Kamenka	Karalana
Julietta	Kaala	Kaikoura	Kalika	Kameo	Karalee
Juliette	Kaara	Kail	Kalila	Kameron	Karalyn
Julina	Kaari	Kaila	Kalin	Kameryn	Karalynn
Julinka	Kaawa	Kailani	Kalina	Kami	Karasi
Julisa	Kaayla	Kailas	Kalinda	Kamiko	Karcsi
Julisha	Kabecka	Kailee	Kalindi	Kamila	Kareena
Juliska	Kabibe	Kailey	Kalisa	Kamilah	Karelma
Julissa	Kabir	Kaili	Kalisfena	Kamili	Karen

91

Karena	Karrie	Katelin	Katreena	Kaylee	Keeisha
Karenza	Karrin	Katelinn	Katrene	Kayleen	Keela
Kari	Karrine	Katell	Katria	Kayleene	Keelan
Karida	Karris	Katelyn	Katriane	Kayleigh	Keeley
Karie	Karryn	Katelynn	Katrice	Kaylen	Keelia
Karima	Karsen	Katen	Katriel	Kaylene	Keelin
Karimah	Karsten	Kateri	Katrien	Kaylenn	Keelty
Karin	Karsyn	Katerina	Katrin	Kaylessa	Keely
Karina	Karuka	Katerinka	Katrina	Kayley	Keelyn
Karinda	Karyme	Katey	Katrine	Kayli	Keemeone
Karine	Karyna	Kathan	Katrinna	Kaylie	Keen
Karinna	Karynn	Katharine	Katrusha	Kayliee	Keena
Karinya	Kasa	Katharyn	Katrya	Kaylin	Keenan
Karis	Kasandra	Katherin	Katryn	Kaylinn	Keenat
Karise	Kasen	Katherina	Katryna	Kaylla	Keenya
Karishma	Kasey	Katherine	Katti	Kayllie	Keeona
Karisma	Kasha	Katherinne	Kattia	Kaylor	Keeran
Kariss	Kashiti	Katheryn	Kattie	Kaylyn	Keerla
Karissa	Kashka	Kathi	Kattina	Kaylynn	Keesha
Karisse	Kashmir	Kathie	Kattrina	Kayson	Keeshia
Karla	Kasi	Kathia	Kattryna	Kayte	Keeton
Karlee	Kasia	Kathleen	Katty	Kayteequa	Keeva
Karleen	Kasiani	Kathleena	Katunia	Kaytie	Keeya
Karleshia	Kasie	Kathlene	Katuscha	Kaywar	Keezheekoni
Karley	Kasienka	Kathlyn	Katy	Kazane	Kefira
Karli	Kaska	Kathlynn	Katya	Kazdoia	Kegan
Karlie	Kasmira	Kathrine	Katyenka	Kazuko	Kei
Karlishia	Kass	Kathryn	Katyushka	Keagan	Keiana
Karlotta	Kassandra	Kathryne	Katyuska	Keaghlan	Keiandra
Karly	Kassia	Kathrynn	Kaula	Keahi	Keiba
Karlyn	Kassiani	Kathy	Kaur	Keaira	Keiki
Karma	Kassidy	Kathya	Kaveri	Keala	Keiko
Karmann	Kassie	Kati	Kavi	Kealii	Keil
Karmel	Kasumi	Katia	Kavindra	Keana	Keila
Karmelita	Kat	Katiana	Kavrala	Keandra	Keilah
Karmen	Kata	Katie	Kawena	Keani	Keilana
Karmia	Katalena	Katima	Kay	Keanna	Keilani
Karmina	Katalin	Katina	Kaya	Keanu	Keir
Karmit	Katalina	Katine	Kayanna	Keara	Keira
Karmiti	Katana	Katinka	Kayce	Kearney	Keirra
Karna	Kataniya	Katinna	Kaycee	Kearra	Keisha
Karol	Katanyna	Katiya	Kayden	Keaton	Keishara
Karolina	Katara	Katja	Kaydence	Keats	Keita
Karoline	Katareena	Katlina	Kayin	Keavy	Keitha
Karoll	Katarina	Katlyn	Kayla	Kedma	Keiyanai
Karoly	Katarzyna	Katlynn	Kaylaa	Keeana	Kelyn
Karpova	Kate	Katniss	Kaylaann	Keeanna	Kekepania
Karpovskaia	Katee	Kato	Kaylah	Keeara	Keladry
Karra	Kateena	Katoka	Kaylana	Keegan	Kelayshia
Karri	Kateisha	Katreen	Kaylann	Keegsquaw	Kelby

Kelcie	Kendria	Kerris	Khayriyya	Kieu	Kimya
Kelcy	Kendrix	Kerry	Kheoniia	Kieve	Kin
Kelda	Kendyl	Kerrya	Khimberly	Kiffany	Kina
Kelemon	Kendyll	Kerryn	Khioniia	Kiffen	Kindle
Kelii	Kenenza	Kerstin	Khloe	Kigva	Kindra
Kelila	Kenia	Kesara	Khlopyreva	Kiho	Kineks
Kelilah	Kenise	Kesare	Khovra	Kiira	Kineret
Kelin	Kenisha	Kesha	Khrana	Kiirsten	Kineta
Kelis	Kenley	Keshet	Khrisiia	Kiisha	Kinfe
Kella	Kenna	Keshia	Khristeen	Kijana	Kinga
Kelleigh	Kenndra	Kesia	Khristen	Kiki	Kingsley
Kellen	Kennedi	Kesley	Khristianova	Kikiliia	Kinipela
Kelley	Kennedy	Kessie	Khristin	Kiku	Kinley
Kelli	Kennice	Ketaki	Khristina	Kilala	Kinnat
Kellie	Kennita	Kethryllia	Khristine	Kilenya	Kinneret
Kellsey	Kennley	Ketifa	Khristyana	Kiley	Kinnette
Kellsi	Kennya	Ketill	Khristyna	Kilikeia	Kinsey
Kellsie	Kensey	Ketura	Khrstina	Kilikiia	Kinsley
Kelly	Kensington	Keturah	Khrystina	Killian	Kinta
Kellyanne	Kensley	Ketzia	Khrystyn	Kim	Kinzie
Kellye	Kentucky	Ketziya	Khrystyna	Kimama	Kiojah
Kellyn	Kenya	Kevay	Khrystyne	Kimana	Kioko
Kelsa	Kenyon	Kevina	Khuong	Kimaya	Kiona
Kelsea	Kenzie	Kevine	Khuyen	Kimba	Kionah
Kelsee	Kenzy	Kevlyn	Khvalibud	Kimbalee	Kione
Kelsei	Keola	Kevyn	Khynika	Kimball	Kioni
Kelsey	Keona	Kew	Kia	Kimber	Kionna
Kelsi	Keonna	Keya	Kiah	Kimberle	Kiora
Kelsie	Kera	Keyah	Kiahna	Kimberlee	Kipling
Kelson	Kerala	Keyanna	Kiana	Kimberley	Kipp
Kelsy	Keran	Keyla	Kiandra	Kimberli	Kiprilla
Keltie	Kerani	Kezia	Kiandria	Kimberlie	Kira
Kelula	Keren	Keziah	Kianga	Kimberlin	Kiraanna
Kelyn	Kerensa	Kfira	Kiani	Kimberlina	Kirabo
Kemberly	Keri	Khadejah	Kiann	Kimberlly	Kiral
Keme	Keriana	Khadiga	Kianna	Kimberly	Kiran
Kemena	Keriann	Khadija	Kianni	Kimberlyn	Kirana
Kemina	Kerianna	Khaleesi	Kiara	Kimberlynn	Kiranda
Kempley	Kerianne	Khalida	Kiaria	Kimberlyy	Kirby
Kenadia	Kerilyn	Khalilah	Kiarra	Kimbra	Kiri
Kenadie	Keris	Khanh	Kiasax	Kimbralcy	Kiriah
Kenda	Kerkıra	Kharesa	Kiauna	Kimeya	Kiriakiia
Kendahl	Kerlisha	Khariessa	Kiba	Kimi	Kiriena
Kendal	Kern	Kharitaniia	Kiden	Kimiko	Kirilla
Kendale	Kerr	Kharitina	Kie	Kimimela	Kirilovskaia
Kendaleigha	Kerra	Kharitona	Kiele	Kimmberly	Kirima
Kendall	Kerri	Kharitonova	Kiera	Kimmie	Kirit
Kendi	Kerrianne	Khatijah	Kieran	Kimmy	Kiros
Kendis	Kerrie	Khayrat	Kierra	Kimn	Kirra
Kendra	Kerrin	Khayri	Kiersten	Kimora	Kirrily

Kirsi	Klynn	Kosa	Krunevichovna	Kuznetsova		**L**
Kirsten	Knikki	Kosenila	Krushka	Kvasena		
Kirstie	Kochava	Kosma	Krysanthe	Kvetava		
Kirstin	Kodi	Kostenka	Krysta	Kwanita		Laamtora
Kirstine	Kodiak	Kostya	Krystal	Kya		Laasya
Kirsty	Kody	Kostyusha	Krystall	Kyan		Labhaoise
Kirtana	Koemi	Kosuke	Krystalyn	Kyden		Laboni
Kirti	Koffi	Kotik	Krysten	Kye		Labonita
Kirya	Kogorshed	Koto	Krystin	Kyla		Lacci
Kisa	Kohaku	Kotone	Krystina	Kylaa		Lace
Kisha	Kohana	Kotono	Krystka	Kylah		Lacee
Kishi	Koia	Kourtney	Krystyn	Kylan		Lacene
Kiska	Koika	Kovan	Krystyna	Kylar		Lacey
Kismet	Koko	Kovana	Ksafipa	Kyle		Laci
Kiss	Kokuro	Kowan	Ksana	Kylee		Laciann
Kissa	Kokyangwuti	Kozakura	Ksanfippa	Kyleigh		Lacie
Kissha	Kolee	Kozma	Ksanochka	Kylene		LaCienega
Kit	Koleyna	Kozmina	Ksena	Kyler		Lacina
Kita	Kolina	Kozue	Ksenia	Kyli		Lacole
Kitena	Kolomianka	Krabava	Kseniia	Kylia		Lacy
Kitkun	Kolton	Krasa	Kseniya	Kylie		Lacyann
Kitoko	Komala	Kreeli	Ksenya	Kyliee		Lada
Kitra	Komali	Krestiia	Kshtovtovna	Kylla		Ladee
Kitron	Kona	Kriendel	Ksnia	Kyllie		Ladonna
Kitsa	Konane	Kris	Ksniatintsa	Kyllii		LaDonna
Kittiana	Konchaka	Krisalyn	Kudra	Kym		Lady
Kitty	Konchasha	Krisandra	Kuma	Kymber		Lael
Kiuprila	Konkordiia	Krishna	Kumani	Kymberlee		Laelia
Kiuriakiia	Konstantiia	Krisstina	Kumba	Kymberli		Laerdya
Kiva	Konstanze	Krista	Kumi	Kymberly		Laetitia
Kivi	Konstiantina	Kristabelle	Kumie	Kymberlyn		Lafayette
Kiwidinok	Konstiantinova	Kristal	Kumiko	Kyna		Laguna
Kiya	Kopin	Kristeen	Kuna	Kyndal		Lahela
Kiyoko	Kora	Kristen	Kunegundy	Kyndall		Lahoma
Kiyoshi	Kordell	Kristian	Kunei	Kyndra		Laia
Kiza	Korene	Kristiana	Kunigunde	Kynlee		Laibah
Kizzy	Koretskaia	Kristiann	Kuniko	Kynthia		Laikina
Kjerstin	Kori	Kristianna	Kunka	Kyo		Laila
Klara	Korina	Kristiina	Kunko	Kyoko		Lailaa
Klarika	Kornelia	Kristin	Kunku	Kyoto		Lailah
Klarissa	Korotkaia	Kristina	Kuntse	Kyou		Laili
Klasha	Korotkova	Kristine	Kura	Kyra		Lailie
Klaudia	Korotsek	Kristinn	Kuri	Kyrah		Laina
Klavdiia	Korotskovaia	Kristinna	Kuriana	Kyrene		Laine
Klavdiya	Korrine	Kristinne	Kuron	Kyria		Lainey
Klee	Kortnee	Kristjana	Kusuma	Kyrie		Lainie
Klementina	Kortney	Kristy	Kuthun	Kyrra		Lair
Kleopatra	Kortni	Kristyn	Kuwanlelenta	Kythaela		Laire
Klotid	Kortnie	Krivulinaia	Kuwanyamtiwa	Kyya		Laisha
Klychikha	Kory	Krizia	Kuwanyauma	Kzhna		Lajita

Lake	Lane	Larra	Laurence	Laylie	Legacy
Lakeesha	Lanee	Larsen	Laurencia	Layna	Legarre
Lakeeshia	Lanelle	Larue	Laurene	Layne	Legend
Lakeisha	Lanetta	Larunda	Laurenn	Laynee	Lehana
Lakeithia	Laney	Larya	Laurentia	Lazziar	Lehava
Lakelyn	Lang	Laryssa	Laurenza	Le	Lei
Laken	Langley	Lashanda	Lauretta	Lea	Leia
Lakendra	Lani	Lasharon	Laurette	Leaf	Leianna
Lakesha	Lanica	Lashunay	Lauriane	Leah	Leigh
Lakessha	Lanice	Lassie	Laurianna	Leahonia	Leigha
Lakia	Lanie	Lata	Laurianne	Leal	Leighann
Lakin	Lanka	Latacia	Laurie	Leala	Leighanna
Lakisha	Lanna	Latanya	Laurien	Lealia	Leighanne
Lakken	Lantana	Latasha	Laurin	Lean	Leighna
Lakota	Lanza	Latassha	Laurinda	Leana	Leighton
Laksha	Laoidheach	Lateefah	Laurissa	Leandra	Leiko
Lakshmi	Laoise	Latiece	Laurita	Leane	Leila
Lakyle	Lapis	Latifa	Laurren	Leann	Leilah
Lala	Lapronda	Latifah	Laurrie	Leanna	Leilani
Lalage	Laqueta	Latika	Laury	Leanndra	Leilanii
Lalaine	Laquinta	Latisha	Lauryn	Leanne	Leilanni
Lalana	Laquisha	Latissha	Laurynn	Leanore	Leilatha
Lalasa	Laquita	Latona	Lavada	Leatrice	Leira
Lalawethika	Lara	Latoya	Lavali	Leatrix	Leire
Laleh	Larae	Latoyya	Lavanda	Lebeau	Leisa
Lalette	Laragh	Latrice	Lavanya	Lecea	Leith
Lali	Laraib	Latricia	Lave	Lechsinska	Lejane
Lalia	Laraine	Latrisha	Laveda	Lecia	Leka
Lalika	Laralaine	Latskaia	Lavender	Leda	Lela
Laline	Laramae	Lauda	LaVergne	Ledah	Leland
Lalita	Laramie	Laudonia	Laverick	Ledell	Lelia
Lalla	Laran	Laufeia	Lavern	Lee	Lelik
Lallie	Laranya	Lauica	Laverna	Leea	Lemuela
Lally	Laras	Laura	Laverne	Leeah	Lena
Lamara	Lareina	Lauraine	Lavernia	Leeandra	Lenae
Lameez	LaReina	Laural	Lavey	Leeann	Lenci
Lamia	Laren	Lauralee	Lavi	Leeanna	Lene
Lamis	Larena	Lauralei	Lavina	Leeanne	Leni
Lamya	Larentia	Lauralie	Lavinia	Leeba	Lenina
Lan	Lari	Lauralyn	Lavonne	Leehi	Lenis
Lana	Laria	Lauran	Lavonte	Leela	Lenka
Lanai	Larina	Laurana	Lawahiz	Leelee	Lenmana
Lanassa	Larinda	Laure	LaWanda	Leena	Lenna
Landa	Larisa	Laureanne	Lawrence	Leeona	Lennon
Landen	Larissa	Laureen	Lawrencia	Leeonna	Lennox
Landra	Larita	Laurel	Laxmi	Leesa	Lenny
Landrada	Lark	Laurelin	Layan	Leesly	Lenochka
Landri	Larkin	Laurella	Laycie	Leester	Lenora
Landry	Larkspur	Laurelle	Layla	Leeto	Lenore
Landyn	Larochka	Lauren	Laylah	Leeza	Lenusy

Lenusya	Leta	Li	Ligaya	Lillybet	Lior
Leocadia	Letesha	Lia	Ligeia	Lilo	Liora
Leocadie	Letha	Liadan	Ligia	Lilou	Lioslaith
Leoda	Lethia	Liama	LiHua	Liluth	Lipa
Leola	Leticia	Lian	Liisa	Liluye	Lira
Leoline	Letisha	Liana	Likla	Lily	Liriene
Leoma	Letitia	Liane	Lil	Lilyana	Lirienne
Leona	Letizia	Lianna	Lila	Lilyanna	Lirit
Leonarda	Letje	Lianne	Lilac	Lilybelle	Lirita
Leonda	Lette	Liat	Lilach	Lilybet	Lis
Leondra	Lettice	Liba	Lilah	Lilybeth	Lisa
Leondrea	Letticia	Libania	Lileas	Limber	Lisabet
Leone	Lettie	Libba	Lili	LiMei	Lisabeth
Leonela	Letty	Libbie	Lilia	LiMing	Lisabette
Leonelle	Letya	Libby	Lilian	Limon	Lisandra
Leonie	Leucothea	Libertad	Liliana	Limor	Lisanka
Leonilla	Leva	Liberty	Liliane	Lin	Lisavet
Leonita	Levana	Libra	Liliann	Lina	Lisaveta
Leonlina	Levane	Libusa	Lilianna	Linaeve	Lisbet
Leonna	Leven	Licia	Lilianne	Linda	Lisbeth
Leonor	Levia	Lida	Lilias	Lindaa	Lise
Leonora	Levina	Lidda	Lilibeth	Linden	Liseetsa
Leonore	Levita	Liddia	Lilie	Lindley	Liseli
Leonteva	Levona	Lidena	Liliha	Lindsay	Liset
Leontien	Levron	Lidewij	Lilika	Lindsee	Liseth
Leontina	Levyna	Lidia	Lilike	Lindsey	Lisette
Leontine	Lewa	Lidiia	Liliosa	Lindsi	Lishka
Leontyne	Lewana	Lidija	Lilis	Lindsie	Lisil
Leopolda	Lewanna	Lidiy	Lilith	Lindsy	Lisimba
Leopoldina	Lex	Lidiya	Liliya	Lindy	Lisinda
Leopoldine	Lexann	Lidka	Lilja	Linette	Liska
Leora	Lexi	Lidmila	Lilka	Ling	Lisle
Leotie	Lexia	Lido	Lilla	Linh	Lisotianka
Lepa	Lexie	Lidocha	Lillah	Linley	Lissa
Lepeka	Lexii	Lidochka	Lilli	Linn	Lissandra
Lequoia	Lexine	Lidwien	Lillia	Linna	Lissbeth
Lera	Lexington	Lidwina	Lillian	Linnda	Lisset
Lerka	Lexis	Liealia	Lilliana	Linnea	Lissette
Leryn	Lexiss	Lieba	Lilliane	Linnet	Lita
Les	Lexus	Lieke	Lilliann	Linnett	Lithany
Lesa	Lexxi	Lien	Lillianna	Linnette	Lithia
Lesham	Lexxie	Liesa	Lillias	Linore	Litzy
Lesia	Lexy	Liesbet	Lillie	Linsey	Liuba
Leslee	Leya	Liesel	Lillis	Linwood	Liubchanina
Lesley	Leyden	Lieselotte	Lillith	Linzee	Liubka
Leslie	Leyla	Liesheth	Lillium	Linzy	Liubokhna
Lesliee	Leyna	Liesl	Lilly	Liolya	Liubone
Leslly	Leysa	Lieu	Lillyana	Lion	Liubov
Lesly	Lezith	Lieve	Lillyann	Liona	Liubusha
Lessly	Lezlie	Liezel	Lillybelle	Lionel	Liudena

Liudmila	Lodema	Lorelle	Louisianna	Lucila	Lunet
Liunharda	Lodima	Loren	Loulou	Lucile	Lunetta
Liutarda	Lodoiska	Lorena	Lourdes	Lucilla	Lunette
Liutsilla	Lodyma	Lorene	Louredes	Lucille	Lunna
Liv	Loe	Lorenia	Louriz	Lucina	Lupe
Livana	Loelia	Lorenn	Louvain	Lucinda	Luperca
Lively	Loften	Lorenna	Louvaine	Lucine	Lupita
Livi	Logan	Lorenza	Lova	Lucita	Lur
Livia	Logestilla	Loreto	Love	Lucja	Lurleen
Livie	Logistilla	Loretta	Lovely	Lucky	Lurline
Livvy	Loida	Lori	Lovelyn	Lucrece	Lusha
Liwanag	Loire	Loria	Lovender	Lucrecia	Lutisha
Lixue	Lois	Lorian	Lovette	Lucretia	Luvena
Liya	Lokelani	Loriana	Lovey	Lucrezia	Luvenia
Liz	Loki	Loriann	Lovie	Lucy	Luvina
Liza	Lol	Lorica	Lovisa	Lucyna	Lux
Lizabeta	Lola	Lorie	Lowri	Luda	Luyu
Lizabeth	Loleta	Loriel	Loyal	Ludiia	Luz
Lizandra	Lolita	Lorii	Loyda	Ludka	Lvovicha
Lizanka	Lolitta	Lorilee	Lualhati	Ludmia	Ly
Lizanne	Lolly	Lorilynn	Luana	Ludmila	Lyalechka
Lizbet	Lolo	Lorin	Luanda	Ludmilla	Lyalya
Lizbeth	Lolovivi	Lorinda	Luba	Ludomia	Lyanna
Lizbethe	Lolya	Loring	Lubachitsa	Ludovica	Lybed
Lizena	Lomahongva	Loris	Lubava	Luella	Lycia
Lizeth	Lomasi	Lorita	Lubmila	Luighseach	Lycoris
Lizette	Lona	Lorna	Lubmilla	Luisa	Lydda
Lizina	London	Lorne	Lubna	Luise	Lyddia
Lizveth	Londyn	Lorra	Lubohna	Luisianna	Lydia
Lizza	Loni	Lorraina	Lubomira	Luiza	Lydian
Lizzbeth	Lonlee	Lorraine	Lubov	Lujayn	Lydie
Lizzie	Lonna	Lorreen	Lubusha	Luka	Lydon
Ljudmila	Lonnie	Lorren	Luca	Lukeria	Lyeta
Ljudmilla	Lonyn	Lorrena	Lucania	Lukerina	Lyla
Llamryl	Lora	Lorretta	Lucasta	Lukerya	Lylah
Llesenia	Lorah	Lorri	Luccia	Lukiia	Lyle
Lleucu	Loraina	Lorrin	Lucciana	Lukina	Lylee
Llinos	Loraine	Lorrina	Lucena	Lukiria	Lylla
Llio	Loralei	Lotta	Lucera	Lukoianova	Lyn
Lluvia	Lorand	Lotte	Lucerne	Lula	Lynae
Lluvy	Lorant	Lottie	Lucero	Lulie	Lynda
Llywelya	Lorayne	Lotus	Lucetta	Lulling	Lynde
Loa	Lorca	Lotye	Lucette	Lulu	Lyndell
Loan	Lorda	Lou	Lucia	Lumen	Lyndon
Loba	Lore	Louanna	Luciana	Lumière	Lyndsay
Lochan	Loreen	Louella	Luciann	Lumina	Lyndsey
Lochana	Loreena	Louisa	Lucianna	Luminita	Lynelle
Lochellen	Lorelai	Louisane	Lucida	Luminosa	Lynessa
Locke	Lorelei	Louise	Lucie	Luna	Lyneth
Locklyn	Lorella	Louisiana	Lucienne	Lundy	Lynette

Lyngheid	Maat	Madalynn	Madisson	Magda	Maialen
Lynlee	Maaya	Madan	Madissyn	Magdala	Maible
Lynley	Maayan	Maddalen	Madisyn	Magdalen	Maida
Lynn	Maaza	Maddalena	Madisynn	Magdalena	Maidel
Lynna	Mab	Maddalyn	Madlaina	Magdalene	Maighdlin
Lynnae	Mabbina	Maddalynn	Madlyn	Magdalia	Maija
Lynnda	Mabel	Maddelena	Madolen	Magdalina	Maiju
Lynndsey	Mabella	Maddeline	Madonna	Magee	Maik
Lynne	Mabelle	Maddelyn	Madora	Magen	Maika
Lynnea	Mabli	Maddelynn	Madra	Magena	Maikki
Lynnell	Mabs	Madden	Madre	Magenta	Maile
Lynnet	Mabyn	Maddie	Madri	Maggen	Maili
Lynnette	Macadrian	Maddisen	Madrid	Maggi	Maille
Lynnsey	Macall	Maddison	Madrigal	Maggie	Maillol
Lynsey	Macarena	Maddisson	Madrona	Maggy	Mailsi
Lynton	Macaria	Maddisyn	Mady	Magic	Mailys
Lynwen	Macaulay	Maddy	Madysen	Magmeteva	Maimun
Lyonette	Macawi	Maddysen	Madyson	Magna	Maina
Lyra	Macayle	Maddyson	Madysson	Magnhilda	Maine
Lyre	Maccaulay	Madeira	Madzeija	Magnild	Maiolaine
Lyric	Macee	Madel	Mae	Magnilda	Mair
Lyrica	Macen	Madelaine	Maeby	Magnilde	Maira
Lyricc	Maceo	Madelein	Maegan	Magnolia	Maire
Lyris	Macey	Madeleina	Maegann	Mago	Mairead
Lysa	Macha	Madeleine	Maeja	Magola	Mairéad
Lysandra	Machara	Madelena	Maeko	Magritte	Mairi
Lysette	Machelle	Madelene	Maela	Maha	Mairia
Lysippe	Machiko	Madelhari	Maelee	Mahah	Mairin
Lysistrata	Machko	Madelia	Maelie	Mahal	Mairona
Lyssa	Machna	Madelief	Maelle	Mahala	Mairwen
Lystra	Maci	Madelin	Maelynn	Mahalah	Maisa
Lyuba	Macie	Madelina	Maelyrra	Mahalia	Maisha
Lyubochka	Maciee	Madeline	Maelys	Mahari	Maisie
Lyubonka	Macii	Madelinne	Maemi	Mahaskah	Maisy
Lyubov	Mackenna	Madelline	Maera	Mahdis	Maita
Lyudmila	Mackenzie	Madellyn	Maeralya	Mahesa	Maitane
Lyudmilla	Maclean	Madelon	Maeron	Mahima	Maite
Lyuha	Macon	Madelyn	Maery	Mahin	Maitea
Lyusya	Maconaquea	Madelynn	Maeryn	Mahina	Maiti
Lyutsiana	Macrae	Madena	Maesen	Mahlah	Maitilda
Lyvia	Macy	Madge	Maeva	Maho	Maitilde
Lyzabeth	Macyn	Madia	Maeve	Mahogany	Maitland
Lyzbeth	Mada	Madie	Mafalda	Mahogony	Maive
	Madailein	Madigan	Magaidh	Mahola	Maiya
M	Madalaine	Madilyn	Magali	Mahsa	Maizah
	Madalen	Madilynn	Magalie	Mahta	Maize
Maaike	Madalena	Madina	Magaly	Mahwah	Maj
Maari	Madalene	Madisen	Magalys	Mai	Maja
Maaria	Madaline	Madison	Magan	Maia	Majella
Maartje	Madalyn	Madissen	Magaska	Maiah	Majesta

Majestas	Maleeah	Malvina	Mao	Marely	Marianela
Majesty	Maleena	Malvinia	Maola	Marelys	Mariangely
Majida	Maleficent	Mame	Maoli	Maremiana	Mariann
Majken	Maleika	Mamelfa	Maolmin	Maren	Marianna
Majorca	Malena	Mami	Maovesa	Marenda	Marianne
Majori	Malencia	Mamie	Maple	Maressa	Marianskaia
Majorie	Malene	Mamika	Mar	Maretta	Mariasha
Makaela	Malgosia	Mana	Mara	Marfa	Mariatu
Makai	Malha	Manae	Marabel	Marfutka	Maribel
Makaila	Mali	Manal	Maraca	Margaid	Maribell
Makaio	Malia	Manami	Marah	Margalit	Maribella
Makala	Maliah	Manasa	Maralah	Margalo	Maribelle
Makalia	Maliha	Mancuso	Maram	Margaret	Maribeth
Makalla	Malika	Manda	Marana	Margareta	Marice
Makana	Malin	Mandala	Maranda	Margarete	Maricel
Makani	Malina	Mandalyn	Maravilla	Margarethe	Maricela
Makara	Malinda	Mandana	Marbella	Margarett	Maricelia
Makawee	Malini	Mandara	Marcail	Margaretta	Maricella
Makayla	Maliny	Mandel	Marcela	Margarita	Maricha
Makaylla	Malisa	Mandelina	Marcelen	Margaux	Marichinich
Makeda	Malise	Mandell	Marcelina	Marge	Maricruz
Makeena	Malissa	Mandi	Marceline	Margeaux	Maridel
Makeiah	Malita	Mandira	Marcella	Marged	Marie
Makelesi	Maliusha	Mandisa	Marcelle	Margeret	Marie-Laure
Makelina	Maliuta	Mandolin	Marcellia	Margerie	Marieke
Makena	Maliyah	Mandoline	Marcellina	Margery	Mariel
Makena'Lei	Malka	Mandy	Marcena	Marggie	Mariela
Makenna	Malka	Manechka	Marcene	Margherita	Mariele
Makenzie	Malkah	Manet	March	Margie	Mariell
Makhna	Malkia	Manette	Marcheline	Margisia	Mariella
Maki	Mallaidh	Mangena	Marchelle	Margit	Marielle
Makimi	Mallia	Mani	Marci	Margita	Marien
Makkitotosimew	Mallika	Manica	Marcia	Margo	Marietta
Makrina	Mallorca	Manika	Marciana	Margolette	Mariette
Maksimina	Malloren	Manila	Marcie	Margolo	Marigold
Maksimova	Mallorie	Manina	Marcy	Margosha	Mariia
Makya	Mallory	Manju	Mardea	Margot	Marija
Mal	Mallow	Manka	Mardella	Margred	Marije
Mala	Malmuira	Manning	Mardi	Margrete	Marijke
Malagueña	Malmuirie	Manoela	Mare	Marguerite	Marika
Malaika	Malona	Manon	Marea	Mari	Marike
Malak	Malonia	Manoush	Maredud	Maria	Mariken
Malana	Malorie	Mansa	Maree	Mariaann	Mariko
Malania	Malou	Mansi	Mareen	Mariabella	Marilee
Malaya	Malruthiia	Manto	Mareena	Mariah	Marilla
Malaysia	Malta	Mantreh	Mareesa	Mariam	Marillyn
Malcah	Malu	Manuela	Mareike	Mariamne	Marilu
Malcolmina	Maluchka	Manya	Marelda	Marian	Marily
Malea	Malusha	Manyiten	Marell	Mariana	Marilyn
Maleah	Malva	Manzie	Marella	Mariane	Marilynn

Marimba	Marjon	Marquesa	Marveille	Materia	Maven
Marimiana	Marjorie	Marquetta	Marvel	Matfeitsa	Maverick
Marin	Marka	Marquette	Marvela	Mathea	Mavis
Marina	Markeisha	Marquilla	Marvell	Mathia	Mavise
Marinda	Markesha	Marquisa	Marvella	Mathild	Mavra
Marine	Markeshia	Marquise	Marvelle	Mathilda	Max
Marinel	Marketa	Marquisha	Marvene	Mathilde	Maxandria
Marinella	Markiana	Marra	Marvina	Mathura	Maxi
Marini	Markie	Marranda	Marwa	Matia	Maxie
Marinka	Markisha	Marren	Mary	Matias	Maxima
Marinn	Markita	Marri	Mary Ann	Matilda	Maxime
Marinna	Marla	Marria	Marya	Matilde	Maxine
Marinochka	Marlaina	Marriah	Maryam	Matisse	Maxwelle
Marinskaia	Marlana	Marriam	Maryan	Mato	May
Marion	Marlas	Marrian	Maryann	Matoaka	Maya
Mariona	Marlayna	Marriana	Maryanna	Matrena	Mayah
Marionilla	Marlee	Marriann	Maryanne	Matriona	Maybeth
Mariota	Marleen	Marrianna	Maryjane	Matrona	Mayda
Mariposa	Marleena	Marrica	Maryl	Matruna	Mayes
Mariquita	Marleene	Marrie	Maryland	Matryona	Maygan
Maris	Marleigh	Marrim	Maryn	Matryoshka	Mayim
Marisa	Marleisha	Marrina	Maryna	Matsuko	Maylasia
Marisabel	Marlen	Marrisa	Maryon	Mattea	Maylee
Marise	Marlena	Marrissa	Maryse	Matthea	Mayleen
Marisela	Marlene	Marry	Marysia	Matthia	Maylene
Marisella	Marlenee	Mars	Maryvonne	Mattie	Mayliesha
Marisha	Marlenne	Marsala	Maryweld	Matty	Maylin
Mariska	Marley	Marsali	Masada	Matuta	Mayme
Marisol	Marli	Marseilles	Masako	Matxalen	Mayra
Marissa	Marlie	Marsh	Masami	Matya	Mayra-Liz
Maristela	Marlin	Marsha	Mascha	Matyidy	Maysa
Marit	Marlina	Marshae	Masha	Matylda	Maysan
Marita	Marline	Marshay	Mashaka	Maud	Maysel
Maritanna	Marlis	Marta	Mashenka	Maude	Maytal
Maritsa	Marlisa	Martainn	Masia	Maura	Mayte
Maritza	Marlise	Marte	Masiel	Maureen	Mayten
Mariuerla	Marlo	Marteena	Masiela	Maurelle	Mayu
Marixa	Marloes	Martemianova	Mason	Maurianne	Mayze
Mariya	Marlow	Martha	Massachusetts	Maurice	Mazal
Mariyah	Marlowe	Marthe	Massey	Maurina	Mazarine
Marja	Marly	Marthine	Massika	Maurine	Mazatl
Marjan	Marlys	Marti	Massima	Maurisa	Mazcho
Marjani	Marmara	Martia	Masumi	Maurissa	Mazel
Marjean	Marna	Martina	Masuyo	Maurizia	Mazhira
Marjeta	Marni	Martine	Matalin	Maury	McKale
Marjka	Marnie	Martinique	Matana	Maurya	Mckayla
Marjo	Marnina	Marufa	Matat	Mausi	McKayla
Marjolaina	Maro	Marulia	Mataya	Mauve	Mckenna
Marjolaine	Marous	Marusya	Matea	Mava	McKenna
Marjolein	Marpesia	Marva	Mateja	Mave	Mckennzie

Mckenzie	Mehira	Melisenda	Mentha	Merona	Michaella
McKinley	Mehitabel	Melisende	Menucha	Merredith	Michaelyn
Mea	Mehitahelle	Melisent	Meoquanee	Merrick	Michal
Meabh	Mehri	Melisha	Meora	Merridy	Michalin
Mead	Mei	Melissa	Mer	Merrigan	Micheala
Meadhbh	Meike	Melissan	Meradee	Merrill	Michela
Meadow	Meiling	Melisssa	Mcralda	Merrily	Michele
Meagan	Meira	Melita	Merav	Merrin	Michelee
Meagann	Meiriona	Melitina	Merce	Merritt	Micheline
Meaghan	Meissa	Melitsa	Merced	Merry	Michella
Meaghann	Meja	Meliza	Mercede	Merryl	Michelle
Meara	Mekaisto	Melka	Mercedees	Merryn	Michellee
Mearr	Mekelle	Mellanie	Mercedes	Mersera	Michellle
Mecca	Mel	Mellina	Mercer	Mertice	Michi
Mechteld	Mela	Mellinda	Merche	Merton	Michie
Meda	Melaina	Mellisa	Merci	Mertysa	Michigan
Medea	Melaine	Mellissa	Mercia	Merveille	Michiko
Medesicaste	Melana	Mellody	Mercilla	Meryl	Michon
Medi	Melanctha	Mellona	Mercina	Meryle	Mickey
Media	Melanee	Melodi	Mercury	Mesa	Micki
Medina	Melaney	Melodie	Mercy	Messiah	Micol
Meditrina	Melangell	Melody	Meredith	Messina	Micole
Medora	Melania	Melora	Meredydd	Meta	Mide
Medrie	Melanie	Melosa	Merel	Metcalf	Midge
Medusa	Melaniia	Melosia	Mererid	Metea	Midha
Meeda	Melanippe	Meltem	Meret	Metta	Midnight
Meegan	Melanne	Melusina	Merete	Mettabel	Midori
Meeghan	Melannie	Melva	Merethyl	Mette	Mieko
Meegwin	Melantha	Melvina	Mergivana	Meyshia	Miesha
Meena	Melanthe	Melynda	Meri	Meztli	Miette
Meera	Melany	Memdi	Meria	Mhina	Mieze
Meg	Melarue	Memengwa	Merialeth	Mi-na	Migdalia
Mega	Melba	Memo	Meriall	Mia	Migina
Megaan	Mele	Memory	Meribah	Miaa	Migisi
Megan	Melecent	Memphis	Merida	Miach	Mignon
Megann	Melena	Mena	Meridel	Miah	Mignonette
Megara	Meletina	Menachema	Meridian	Miakoda	Miguela
Megdn	Meli	Menachemah	Meriel	Miami	Mihewi
Meggan	Melia	Mendi	Merilee	Miata	Miho
Megghan	Melicent	Mendie	Merilyn	Mica	Miia
Meggie	Meliffany	Mendota	Merinda	Micaela	Miika
Meggy	Melika	Menefer	Meris	Micaella	Miina
Meghaan	Melina	Menemsha	Merise	Micah	Mika
Meghan	Melinda	Meng	Merkaba	Mical	Mikaela
Meghana	Melinna	Menglad	Merkureva	Micha	Mikaella
Meghann	Meliora	Menna	Merla	Michael	Mikaia
Meguinis	Melisa	Menora	Merlara	Michaela	Mikara
Megumi	Melisaa	Menshikova	Merle	Michaele	Mikayla
Mehera	Melisande	Mensonsea	Merlyn	Michaelina	Mikaylla
Meheytabel	Mélisande	Mentari	Merna	Michaeline	Mikele

Mikelle	Milla	Minodora	Mirracle	Mladris	Monnica
Mikey	Millay	Minoo	Mirranda	Mliss	Monone
Mikhaila	Milleise	Minor	Mirre	Mnuvae	Monroe
Mikhailova	Miller	Minorca	Mirren	Mo	Monserrat
Miki	Milley	Minou	Mirta	Moa	Montana
Mikiesha	Millicent	Minowa	Mirte	Moana	Monti
Mikil	Millicente	Mint	Mirtha	Moanna	Montserrat
Mikitina	Millie	Minta	Miruna	Mobley	Montsho
Mikka	Mills	Minty	Misa	Mocha	Mony
Mikkayla	Milly	Minuet	Misae	Modesta	Moody
Mikkel	Milne	Minuit	Misaki	Modeste	Moon
Mikki	Milohna	Minya	Mischa	Modesty	Moona
Mikko	Milokhna	Mio	Misericordia	Modlen	Moonlight
Miku	Miloslava	Mira	Misha	Moe	Mopsa
Mikula	Milou	Mirabel	Missa	Moesha	Mor
Mikulina	Miloushka	Mirabella	Mississippi	Mohala	Mora
Mila	Miluska	Mirabelle	Missouri	Moibeal	Morag
Milaan	Mim	Miracle	Missty	Moiko	Mórag
Milada	Mimi	Mirage	Missy	Moina	Moral
Milagra	Mimir	Mirah	Mist	Moira	Morava
Milagritos	Mimis	Miranda	Mista	Moire	Morawa
Milagros	Mimosa	Mirannda	Mistelee	Moireach	Morcan
Milagrosa	Min	Mirari	Misti	Moise	More
Milakhna	Mina	Mircea	Mistico	Mojgan	Moreen
Milan	Minaal	Mireia	Mistie	Moke	Morela
Milana	Minah	Mireille	Mistique	Molara	Morella
Milandu	Minako	Mireio	Misty	Molli	Morena
Milania	Minal	Mirel	Misu	Mollie	Morey
Milata	Minali	Mirele	Mita	Molly	Morgaine
Milava	Minami	Mirella	Mitali	Momoka	Morgan
Milcah	Minda	Mirelle	Mitena	Momoko	Morgana
Mildred	Mindel	Miren	Mitra	Mona	Morgandy
Milehva	Mindie	Mirena	Mitrodora	Monaco	Morgane
Milekha	Mindy	Mirette	Mitsis	Monahan	Morgann
Milena	Minerva	Mireya	Mitsu	Monaique	Morgant
Milenia	Minetta	Miri	Mitsuko	Monalisa	Morgause
Milesa	Minette	Miriam	Mitzi	Monca	Morgayne
Mileva	Ming	Mirian	Miu	Moncha	Morgwais
Miley	Ming Lee	Mirielle	Miuccia	Monchonsia	Moria
Mili	MingYue	Mirilla	Miwa	Monday	Moriah
Milia	Minh	Mirin	Miya	Monet	Morice
Miliana	Miniona	Mirinda	Miyako	Monica	Moriel
Miliani	Miniya	Mirit	Miyanda	Monifa	Moriko
Milica	Minjonet	Mirla	Miyo	Monika	Morisa
Miliia	Minka	Miró	Miyoko	Moniqua	Morise
Milika	Minna	Mironova	Miyu	Monique	Morissa
Mililani	Minnehaha	Miropiia	Mizell	Monisha	Morit
Militsa	Minnesota	Miroslava	Mizinovskaia	Monissa	Morley
Milja	Minnie	Mirozlava	Mizuki	Monita	Morna
Milka	Minny	Mirra	Mlada	Monkaushka	Morning

Moroccan	Mulan	Mylla	Nadia	Nakeisha	Naroa
Morocco	Mumina	Myma	Nadida	Nakia	Narva
Morowa	Muna	Myra	Nadie	Nakiasha	Nascha
Morriah	Muncel	Myranda	Nadine	Nakita	Nasha
Morrigan	Muniia	Myrella	Nadira	Nakkia	Nashawna
Morrin	Munin	Myrelle	Nadiya	Nakotah	Nashira
Morrisa	Muniya	Myriam	Nadja	Nala	Nashota
Morrisania	Munro	Myriani	Nadjenka	Nalani	Nashua
Morrison	Munya	Myrilla	Nadra	Nalanie	Nashwa
Morticia	Mura	Myrina	Nadusha	Nalda	Nasia
Morven	Murel	Myrla	Nadya	Nallely	Nasim
Morvudd	Murgatroyd	Myrna	Nadyenka	Nambra	Nasima
Morwen	Muriel	Myrra	Nadysha	Namid	Nasira
Morwenna	Muroniia	Myrrh	Nadyuiska	Nampeyo	Nasnan
Morwyn	Murphy	Myrtle	Nadzia	Nan	Nasrin
Moryggan	Murran	Myshka	Naeva	Nana	Nastaran
Mose	Murray	Myslna	Naevys	Nancey	Nastasia
Moselle	Murron	Mystery	Nafisa	Nanci	Nastasich
Mosi	Muse	Mystique	Naflah	Nancie	Nastasiia
Mosley	Musetta	Mystral	Nafuna	Nancsi	Nastasja
Mostyn	Musette	Mythili	Nagida	Nancy	Nastassia
Moto	Music	Mythri	Naglaya	Nanelia	Nastenka
Mouna	Musidora	Myya	Nahal	Nanelle	Nastia
Mounya	Muskan		Nahara	Nanette	Nastiona
Mousia	Musoke	**N**	Nahla	Nani	Nastionka
Mowanza	Mut		Nahlah	Nanine	Nastiusha
Mowway	Muta	Na'Kesha	Nahuatl	Nann	Nastka
Moxie	Mutia	Naadia	Naia	Nanna	Nasya
Moya	Muza	Naama	Naiara	Nannette	Nat
Moyna	My	Naamah	Naida	Nannie	Nata
Mozyr	Mya	Naamit	Naiima	Nanny	Natachia
Mpho	Myaa	Naara	Naila	Nanon	Natacia
Mrinal	Myah	Naarah	Nailah	Nantale	Natala
Mstislava	Mychal	Naava	Nailea	Nanthleene	Natale
Mstislavliaia	Mychele	Naavah	Naima	Naoko	Natalee
Mu	Mychelle	Nabila	Nainsi	Naomi	Natalia
Muadhnait	Myee	Nabirye	Nairi	Naomii	Natalie
Mubina	Myeisha	Nada	Nairna	Napia	Nataliee
Mucia	Myesha	Nadalia	Nairne	Napua	Natalii
Mudri	Myeshia	Nadda	Nairobi	Nara	Nataliia
Muerlara	Myfanawy	Nadeek	Naiser	Narcisa	Natalija
Mufaddal	Myfanwy	Nadeekovaia	Naiya	Narcissa	Natalja
Mugisa	Myisha	Nadeen	Naja	Narcisse	Natalka
Muguet	Myla	Nadege	Najah	Narda	Natallia
Muira	Mylaela	Nadejda	Najia	Narella	Natallie
Muire	Mylaerla	Nadenka	Najiba	Naretha	Natally
Muireann	Mylan	Nadetta	Najila	Nariko	Nataly
Muirgen	Mylee	Nadette	Najinca	Narissa	Natalya
Muirgheal	Myles	Nadezda	Najla	Narkissa	Natana
Muirne	Mylie	Nadezhda	Najwa	Narnia	Natane

103

Natania	Nawa	Nefertiti	Neomenia	Neves	Nik
Nataniela	Nawra	Nefisa	Neomi	Neviah	Nika
Natara	Nay	Nefret	Neomonni	Nevis	Nike
Natascha	Naya	Negeen	Neona	Newlyn	Nikeesha
Natasha	Nayan	Neha	Neonila	Neylan	Nikeiza
Natashaly	Nayana	Nehama	Neorah	Neza	Niki
Natashenka	Nayara	Nehara	Nephele	Nezhatok	Nikiforova
Natashia	Nayeli	Neil	Nephthys	Nezhdakha	Nikita
Natashya	Nayely	Neila	Neptune	Nezhka	Nikitina
Natasia	Nayo	Neilina	Nera	Ngaio	Nikitta
Natassha	Naysa	Neima	Nere	Ngozi	Nikki
Natassia	Nazaret	Neith	Nerea	Nia	Nikkii
Natesa	Nazarova	Neiva	Nereida	Niabi	Nikkita
Nathaira	Nazelli	Nejma	Nereyda	Niagara	Nikkitta
Nathalee	Nazira	Neka	Nergui	Niall	Nikkol
Nathalia	Nazli	Nekana	Neri	Niamh	Nikkylia
Nathalie	Nazneen	Nekane	Neria	Niani	Niko
Nathally	Nazy	Nekoda	Neriah	Niara	Nikolena
Nathaly	Nea	Nekrasa	Nerice	Nica	Nikolia
Nathania	Neal	Nekrasia	Nerida	Nicanora	Nikolina
Nathara	Neala	Nelda	Neried	Nicasia	Niksha
Nathari	Nealie	Nelia	Nerilla	Nicci	Nila
Nathasha	Nealy	Nelida	Nerina	Niccola	Nilda
Nathifa	Nebracha	Neliuba	Nerine	Niccole	Nile
Nathifah	Nebraga	Nelka	Nerissa	Nichelle	Nilea
Natia	Nebraska	Nelke	Nerita	Nichol	Niley
Natie	Nebula	Nell	Nerola	Nichole	Nili
Natine	Nechama	Nella	Nery	Nicholle	Nilima
Natividad	Neci	Nellary	Nerys	Nicia	Nilla
Natsu	Necia	Nellie	Nesdits	Nickelle	Nilou
Natsuki	Neda	Nellis	Nesha	Nicki	Niloufer
Natsuko	Nedaa	Nellwyn	Nesiah	Nico	Nilsine
Natsumi	Nedana	Nelly	Nessa	Nicola	Nima
Nattalie	Nedda	Nelma	Nessia	Nicole	Nimah
Nattaly	Nedelia	Nelsey	Nessie	Nicolee	Nimai
Natuche	Nedelya	Nemea	Nesta	Nicoletta	Nimat
Natura	Nediva	Nemera	Nesy	Nicolette	Nimeesha
Nature	Nedivah	Nemesis	Net	Nicolina	Nimfodora
Naumys	Nedra	Nemilka	Neta	Nicoline	Nimra
Naunet	Neeja	Nemka	Netis	Nicolle	Nin
Nauricia	Neel	Nemy	Netka	Nicosia	Nina
Nausicaa	Neela	Nena	Netta	Nidia	Ninacska
Nautica	Neele	Neneca	Nettie	Nieve	Ninarika
Nava	Neeltje	Nenet	Neued	Nieves	Ninel
Naveen	Neely	Nenetl	Neva	Nifantova	Ninetta
Naveena	Neema	Nenna	Nevada	Nigella	Ninette
Navi	Neena	Neo	Nevaeh	Nighean	Ninfa
Navit	Neenah	Neola	Nevara	Nighinn	Ning
Navy	Neesha	Neoma	Neve	Niia	Ninian
Navya	Nefertari	Neomea	Neveah	Nijlon	Ninna

104

Ninockha	Noelle	Norrah	Nya	Ochyllyss	Ohanna
Ninon	Noely	Norris	Nyah	Octavia	Ohara
Ninotchka	Noemi	North	Nyakio	October	Ohawna
Niobe	Noemie	Nostasia	Nyako	Oda	Ohela
Nira	Noga	Notchimine	Nyala	Odahingum	Ohio
Niria	Nogah	Notin	Nyasia	Odalys	Ohtli
Nirit	Nohealani	Nouf	Nyathera	Odanda	Oifa
Nirvana	Nokomis	Nour	Nydia	Oddveig	Oihane
Nisa	Nola	Noura	Nyeki	Ode	Oilbhe
Nisha	Nolan	Nouvel	Nyimbo	Odeda	Olwyna
Nishelle	Noland	Nova	Nyla	Odede	Ojai
Nishi	Nolcha	Novalee	Nylaa	Odele	Ojal
Nisi	Noleta	Novea	Nylaathria	Odeletta	Okal
Nissa	Nolita	November	Nylah	Odelette	Okalani
Nisse	Nolwenn	Novia	Nylla	Odelia	Okapi
Nita	Noma	Nowles	Nympha	Odell	Oke
Nitara	Nomalanga	Nox	Nynette	Odella	Okena
Nitasha	Nomasonto	Noxolo	Nyofu	Odelya	Oki
Nitca	Nomatha	Noy	Nyoka	Odera	Okinfieva
Nitsa	Nomble	Noya	Nyomi	Odessa	Oklahoma
Nittawosew	Nomi	Nozomi	Nyree	Odetta	Okoth
Nituna	Nomuula	Nsombi	Nysa	Odette	Oksana
Nitya	Non	Nu	Nyssa	Odgerel	Oksanna
Nitza	Nona	Nuala	Nysse	Odiana	Oksanochka
Nitzan	Nonn	Nualla	Nyura	Odiane	Okseniia
Nitzana	Nonna	Nubia	Nyusha	Odigitriia	Oksinia
Nitzanah	Nonnie	Nueleth	Nyx	Odila	Oksiutka
Niva	Noor	Nuha		Odile	Oktyabrina
Nivritti	Noora	Nuhad	**O**	Odilia	Okulina
Nixi	Noorah	Nuin		Odin	Ola
Nixie	Nora	Nukpana	O'Brien	Odina	Olabisi
Nixzaliz	Noraa	Numees	O'Keeffe	Odintsova	Olademis
Niyati	Norabel	Nuna	Oak	Odonna	Olaniyi
Nizana	Norah	Nunekhiia	Oakes	Odra	Olathe
Njema	Noralie	Nunzia	Oakley	Odysseia	Olava
Nkechi	Norbeta	Nuovis	Oana	Ofce	Olea
Nlaea	Nordica	Nur	Oanez	Ofelia	Oleander
Nneke	Noreen	Nura	Oba	Ofimia	Olechka
Nnena	Noreena	Nuray	Obama	Ofira	Oleisa
Nnenia	Norell	Nureet	Obedience	Ofra	Oleisia
Noa	Nori	Nuri	Obelia	Ogafia	Oleksandra
Noah	Noriko	Nuria	Oberon	Ogafitsa	Olena
Nocturna	Norina	Nurit	Obioma	Ogashka	Olencia
Noe	Norine	Nurita	Obrezkova	Ogenya	Olenitsa
Noel	Norma	Nurrin	Ocarina	Ogin	Olenka
Noelani	Normaa	Nuru	Ocean	Ografena	Olenna
Noele	Normandie	Nusa	Oceana	Ogrifina	Olesia
Noelia	Normandy	Nushala	Oceane	Ogrofena	Olesya
Noell	Norna	Nusi	Oceanna	Ogrufena	Oleta
Noella	Norra	Nuttah	Ocheckka	Ogrufina	Olethea

Olexa	Onaona	Orela	Orsha	Ovdokea	Paley
Olfereva	Onawa	Orella	Orshinaia	Ovdotia	Palika
Olga	Ondine	Orenda	Orsina	Ovdotitsa	Palila
Olginitsa	Ondrea	Orenka	Orsola	Ove	Palin
Olgirdovna	Ondreiana	Orfea	Orszebet	Overton	Pall
Olgov	Oneida	Orghlaith	Ortal	Ovidia	Pallas
Oliana	Onella	Ori	Ortemeva	Ovtsa	Pallavi
Olicia	Oneonta	Oria	Ortensia	Owen	Palma
Olida	Oni	Oriana	Orthia	Owena	Palmira
Olimpiada	Onida	Orianna	Ortygia	Owethu	Paloma
Olina	Onit	Orianthe	Orva	Ownah	Palomina
Olinda	Onnjel	Oribella	Orya	Oxana	Pam
Oline	Ono	Orida	Orzora	Oxide	Pamela
Olisa	Onora	Oriel	Orzsebet	Oya	Pamelia
Olisava	Onoslava	Orien	Osaka	Oyintsa	Pamella
Olita	Ontonia	Orina	Osana	Oz	Pamina
Olive	Ontsiforova	Orinda	Osane	Ozanka	Pammela
Olivera	Ontsyforova	Orino	Osanna	Ozara	Pamuy
Oliveria	Onyx	Orinthia	Osceola	Ozma	Panama
Olivette	Oona	Oriole	Osipova		Panchali
Olivia	Oonagh	Orion	Osliabia	**P**	Pandara
Olivie	Ootadabun	Orit	Osma		Pandita
Olkha	Opa	Orla	Osnat	Pabla	Pandora
Olla	Opal	Orlaith	Ostafia	Paccia	Pandra
Olle	Opaline	Orlanda	Ostankova	Pace	Panfilova
Ollive	Opel	Orlantha	Ostashkova	Pacey	Pangiota
Ollivia	Opera	Orleanna	Ostia	Paciencia	Pania
Oluchi	Ophelia	Orleans	Oswalda	Pacifica	Paniz
Olufemi	Ophelie	Orlee	Osyenya	Padget	Panna
Olwen	Ophira	Orlena	Osyka	Padma	Panphila
Olwina	Ophra	Orlenda	Otamisia	Padme	Pansemna
Olwyn	Ophrah	Orlene	Othelia	Pagan	Pansy
Olya	Oprah	Orli	Otrera	Page	Panteha
Olympe	Oprosiniia	Orlina	Ottaline	Pahana	Panthea
Olympia	Ora	Orlitza	Ottavia	Pahukumaa	Pantislava
Olyvia	Orabella	Orly	Ottelien	Paige	Pantyslawa
Olzhbeta	Oracia	Orma	Otthild	Paili	Panya
Oma	Orah	Ormanda	Ottilia	Paislee	Panyin
Omah	Oralee	Orna	Ottilie	Paisley	Paola
Omaira	Orali	Ornella	Ottillia	Paiton	Paolina
Omarosa	Oralia	Ornetta	Ottoline	Paityn	Papatya
Omat	Oralie	Ornice	Otylia	Paiva	Paphos
Omega	Orane	Ororo	Otzara	Paki	Papina
Omelfa	Orange	Orpah	Ouida	Pakuna	Paprika
Omette	Oratilwe	Orphea	Ouisa	Pakwa	Paquita
Ominotago	Orbona	Orquidea	Ouray	Paladia	Paraaha
Omorose	Orchid	Orquidia	Outacite	Palantina	Paradice
Omyra	Ordell	Orra	Ova	Palasha	Paradisa
Ona	Orea	Orrtha	Ovdeeva	Palba	Paramona
Onaiwah	Oreen	Orsa	Ovdiukha	Palesa	Paras

Parasha	Paulette	Pele	Petah	Phoebe	Pippi
Parasia	Paulille	Pelia	Petal	Phoebee	Pirate
Paraskova	Paulina	Pella	Petaluma	Phoena	Piri
Paraskovga	Pauline	Penarddun	Petra	Phoenice	Pirueva
Paraskovgiia	Paulita	Penelope	Petrina	Phoenix	Pisces
Paraskovia	Paulla	Penina	Petronela	Phoenixx	Pistol
Paraskoviia	Paullina	Peninah	Petronella	Phuingara	Pitina
Parastoo	Pauwau	Penna	Petronelle	Phuong	Pixi
Paratyl	Pavana	Pennelope	Petronia	Phylicia	Pixie
Parca	Pavati	Penny	Petronila	Phyliss	Pixii
Pari	Pavel	Penrose	Petronilla	Phyllicia	Pizi
Pariis	Pavla	Pensee	Petronille	Phyllida	Placenta
Paris	Pavlova	Penthea	Petrova	Phyllis	Placida
Parisa	Pavloveia	Penthia	Petrovna	Phynley	Placidia
Parker	Pavlusha	Peony	Petsa	Phyre	Plakida
Parmenia	Pax	Pepita	Petula	Phyrra	Platonida
Parnella	Paxton	Pepper	Petulia	Pia	Pleasance
Paroskova	Payge	Perchta	Petunia	Piaf	Pleasant
Parrish	Payne	Percy	Peyton	Piala	Pleiade
Parthenia	Payson	Perdita	Peza	Piama	Pleuntje
Parthenope	Payton	Peredeslava	Phaedra	Piapot	Plum
Parvati	Paytton	Peregrine	Phaerl	Piav	Pluto
Pascala	Paz	Perfecta	Phedora	Picabia	Pnina
Pascale	Paza	Peri	Phedra	Picabo	Po
Pascaline	Pazia	Peridot	Phelorna	Piccolo	Pocahontas
Pasclina	Paziah	Perke	Phemia	Piedad	Poe
Pascoe	Pazice	Perkhta	Pheobe	Pier	Poesy
Pascua	Pazit	Perkhte	Pheodora	Piera	Poet
Pasha	Pchuneia	Perla	Pherenike	Pierce	Poetry
Pastora	Peace	Permelia	Phiala	Pierette	Pokinaria
Pat	Peaches	Pernella	Phila	Pierina	Pola
Patches	Peachy	Pernilla	Philadelphia	Pierretta	Poladia
Patia	Peale	Pero	Philana	Pierrette	Polazhitsa
Patience	Pearl	Perouze	Philantha	Pieta	Polexia
Patientia	Pearla	Perpetua	Philberta	Pietra	Polia
Patriccia	Pearle	Perpetuia	Philena	Piina	Polikseniia
Patrice	Pearlina	Perri	Philiberta	Pilar	Polikwaptiwa
Patricia	Pechta	Perrin	Philida	Pili	Polina
Patriciaa	Pecola	Perrine	Philippa	Pilialoha	Polinaria
Patrizia	Pedra	Perry	Philippina	Pilis	Poliuzhaia
Patrova	Pedrine	Persephone	Philippine	Pillan	Poll
Patrricia	Peg	Persephonie	Philis	Pilot	Polly
Patsy	Pegeen	Persia	Phillida	Pima	Pollyanna
Patti	Peggy	Persis	Phillipa	Piminova	Poloma
Pattricia	Peigi	Peru	Philomela	Ping	Poloneika
Patty	Pelaga	Perzsi	Philomena	Pink	Polotsk
Patzi	Pelageia	Perzsike	Philomina	Piper	Polotska
Paula	Pelageya	Pesha	Philopena	Piperel	Poloudnitsa
Paulana	Pelagia	Pessa	Philothea	Pippa	Polovinova
Paule	Pelagiia	Peta	Philyra	Pipper	Pomeline

107

Pomme	Priba	Purity	Quirina	Radosta	Rainbow
Pomnislavka	Pribyslava	Puteshineia	Quirtsquip	Radoste	Raine
Pomona	Priela	Putok	Quita	Radozte	Rainelle
Pompliia	Priia	Putokoveia	Quoba	Radslava	Rainey
Ponaria	Prikseda	Putri	Quynh	Rae	Rainie
Pooja	Prima	Pyrene	Qwara	Raeanne	Rainna
Popliia	Primavera		Qwin	Raechel	Rainy
Popo	Primrose	**Q**		Raee	Raisa
Popova	Primula		**R**	Raegan	Raisel
Poppy	Princess	Qadira		Raegann	Raisie
Porcelain	Prisca	Qeturah	Raaina	Raejiisa	Raison
Poroskova	Priscila	Qiana	Raakel	Raelyn	Raissa
Porsche	Priscilla	Qianna	Raanana	Raelynn	Raiza
Porsha	Priskilla	Qianru	Raananah	Raerauntha	Raizel
Porter	Priskula	Qiturah	Raaya	Raeven	Raja
Portia	Prissy	Quadeisha	Rabab	Raewyn	Rajani
Poseanye	Prita	Quamara	Rabah	Rafa	Rajiya
Posey	Priti	Quana	Rabanne	Rafaela	Rajna
Posh	Priya	Quanda	Rabea	Rafela	Rakeem
Posy	Priyanka	Quarry	Rabia	Raffaela	Rakel
Potina	Proksha	Quartilla	Rabiah	Raffaella	Rakhiel
Poved	Promise	Queen	Rach	Rafferty	Raleigh
Povitamun	Proniakina	Queena	Rachael	Rafika	Ralphina
Poviyemo	Prophetess	Queenie	Rachana	Rafiki	Rama
Powaqa	Prosdoka	Queeny	Rachel	Rafiqa	Ramana
Powasheek	Proskudiia	Quela	Rachele	Rafiya	Ramilah
Prairie	Prosper	Quella	Rachell	Raga	Ramira
Praise	Prospera	Quenby	Rachelle	Ragine	Ramla
Praskovja	Provence	Quenna	Rachna	Ragnara	Ramona
Praskovya	Pru	Querida	Racquel	Ragneda	Ramsay
Praxis	Prudence	Questa	Racquell	Ragnhild	Ramya
Prebrana	Prudencia	Queta	Rada	Ragni	Ran
Precia	Prune	Quiana	Radella	Ragnild	Rana
Preciosa	Prunella	Quianna	Radeyah	Ragnilde	Ranae
Precious	Prunellie	Quibilah	Radha	Ragosna	Randa
Predslava	Przhibislava	Quies	Radhiya	Rahat	Randee
Predyslava	Przybyslawa	Quieta	Radia	Rahel	Randi
Preia	Psyche	Quilla	Radiah	Rahele	Randie
Preksedys	Pua	Quinby	Radinka	Rahil	Randilyn
Prema	Puck	Quince	Radivilovna	Rahima	Randy
Premala	Puebla	Quincey	Radka	Rahimat	Rane
Premislava	Pukhleriia	Quincy	Radmila	Rahiq	Ranee
Prentice	Pules	Quinlan	Radmilla	Rahma	Rani
Prepedigna	Pulkheriia	Quinn	Rado	Rai	Rania
Presencia	Puma	Quinta	Radok	Raia	Ranice
Presley	Puna	Quintana	Radokhna	Raicheal	Ranielle
Press	Pura	Quintessa	Radokovaia	Raidah	Ranit
Presta	Pureza	Quintessence	Radonia	Raimunda	Ranita
Presthlava	Purificacion	Quintia	Radosha	Rain	Raniya
Preston	Purisima	Quintina	Radoslava	Raina	Raniyah

108

Ranjana	Raysel	Regina	Rennie	Rhondda	Rilian
Rannveig	Rayven	Regine	Rennie	Rhonwen	Rilla
Ransom	Rayya	Reginna	Renny	Rhoslyn	Rille
Ranya	Raz	Reginy	Renske	Rhoswen	Rima
Raoghnailt	Razi	Rehan	Reseda	Rhosyn	Rimba
Raonaid	Razia	Rei	Reshunda	Rhya	Rimma
Raoule	Raziah	Reia	Reta	Rhynisha	Rimon
Raphaela	Raziela	Reicza	Retta	Rhys	Rimona
Raphaella	Razili	Reid	Reuel	Rhythm	Rin
Rapture	Raziya	Reign	Reuelle	Ria	Rina
Raquel	Rea	Reignbeau	Reut	Rialta	Rinah
Raquell	Reading	Reignbow	Reva	Riana	Rinda
Rasha	Reagan	Reihan	Revanche	Riane	Rineke
Rashanda	Reagann	Reika	Reveka	Rianna	Rini
Rashida	Reaghan	Reiki	Revel	Rianne	Rinna
Rashika	Reanna	Reiko	Reverie	Rica	Rinnah
Rasia	Reba	Reilly	Revital	Ricadonna	Rio
Rasida	Rebbeca	Reina	Revonda	Ricarda	Rioghnach
Rasima	Rebbecca	Reine	Rexanne	Ricci	Riona
Rasine	Rebeca	Reinette	Rey	Richael	Ripley
Ratana	Rebecaa	Reinna	Reya	Richarda	Ripsimia
Rathiain	Rebecal	Réka	Reyn	Richca	Risa
Rathnait	Rebecca	Rekha	Reyna	Richelle	Risha
Rathtyen	Rebekah	Rella	Reynold	Richica	Rishelle
Ratih	Rebekka	Relyea	Rez	Richika	Rishi
Ratka	Rebekkah	Remarkable	Reza	Richikha	Rishona
Ratslava	Rebel	Remedios	Rhan	Richtca	Rislava
Raveen	Rechkina	Remedy	Rhapsody	Richza	Rissa
Raveena	Red	Remember	Rhawn	Ricki	Rita
Raven	Reda	Remi	Rhaxma	Rickie	Ritsa
Ravenna	Reddi	Memmi	Rhea	Rickki	Ritta
Ravid	Reddie	Remmie	Rheanna	Rida	Riva
Ravin	Redeemer	Remy	Rhedyn	Rider	Rivage
Ravyn	Redell	Ren	Rheta	Ridley	Rive
Rawiya	Ree	Rena	Rhetta	Ridwana	River
Rawnie	Reece	Renae	Rheya	Rigg	Rivera
Rawya	Reed	Renaee	Rhiain	Rigmor	Riviera
Ray	Reegan	Renana	Rhian	Rigmora	Rivka
Raya	Reem	Renata	Rhianna	Rigny	Riya
Rayan	Reena	Renate	Rhiannon	Rihana	Rizwana
Rayann	Reese	Rene	Rhianu	Rihanna	Rizzo
Raydeisha	Reeta	Renee	Rhianwen	Riia	Roan
Raylan	Reeve	Renée	Rhianwyn	Riina	Roana
Raylyn	Refiye	Renesmee	Rhoda	Rika	Roann
Raymonda	Refugia	Renessa	Rhodanthe	Rikka	Roanna
Rayna	Regan	Renestrae	Rhodes	Rikki	Robbi
Rayne	Regann	Renita	Rhodos	Rikku	Robbia
Raynee	Reggan	Renitta	Rhody	Riko	Robbin
Raynna	Reggie	Renna	Rhona	Riksa	Robbyn
Raynne	Reggina	Rennae	Rhonda	Riley	Robena

Roberta	Ronaele	Rosanna	Rowanne	Rune	Sabetha
Robertia	Ronalda	Rosanne	Rowdy	Runisha	Sabia
Robertta	Ronalee	Rosaria	Rowena	Rupali	Sabina
Robijn	Ronat	Rosario	Roxana	Ruqayyah	Sabine
Robin	Ronda	Rosary	Roxane	Ruri	Sable
Robina	Rondell	Roscislawa	Roxanna	Rusa	Sabra
Robinetta	Ronela	Roscoe	Roxanne	Ruslana	Sabreen
Robinette	Ronelle	Rose	Roxie	Rusna	Sabreena
Robinn	Ronelyn	Rose Marie	Roxy	Russet	Sabrena
Robyn	Ronen	Roseann	Roy	Russia	Sabri
Robynn	Rong	Roseanna	Roya	Rusti	Sabriel
Roch	Roni	Roseanne	Royal	Rusty	Sabrina
Rochelle	Ronia	Roseclere	Royale	Rut	Sabrinna
Rocio	Ronit	Roselaine	Royanna	Ruta	Sabriyya
Rocket	Roniya	Roselle	Royce	Ruth	Sabryna
Roderica	Ronja	Rosellen	Roz	Ruthann	Sacagawea
Roderiga	Ronli	Roselyn	Roza	Ruwa	Sacajawea
Roesia	Ronna	Roselynn	Rozalia	Ruya	Sacha
Rogelyn	Ronnda	Rosemarie	Rozamond	Ruzgar	Sachet
Rogena	Ronni	Rosemarry	Rozemarijn	Ryan	Sachi
Rogene	Ronnie	Rosemary	Rozene	Ryane	Sachiko
Rogned	Ronny	Rosemond	Rozgneda	Ryann	Sada
Rohais	Roos	Rosemonde	Rozhneva	Ryatt	Sadaf
Rohan	Roosje	Rosemunda	Rozyuka	Ryder	Sadah
Rohana	Roosmarijn	Rosetta	Ruana	Rylan	Sadbh
Roial	Roro	Rosette	Ruba	Ryland	Saddie
Rois	Rory	Roshan	Rubaina	Rylea	Sade
Roisin	Ros	Roshni	Rubby	Rylee	Sadee
Roja	Rosa	Rosie	Rubena	Ryleigh	Sadhbba
Roksana	Rosabel	Rosina	Rubi	Rylen	Sadhbh
Rolanda	Rosabella	Rosine	Rubie	Rylie	Sadia
Roldana	Rosae	Rosita	Rubrae	Ryliee	Sadie
Roline	Rosalba	Rositsa	Ruby	Ryllae	Sadiee
Rollin	Rosalee	Roslyn	Ruchama	Ryllie	Sadiki
Roma	Rosaleen	Roslava	Ruchira	Ryo	Sadira
Romaine	Rosalia	Roslyn	Rudelle	Ryska	Sadiya
Romana	Rosalie	Ross	Rudi		Saelihn
Romane	Rosalina	Rossa	Rudy	**S**	Saeran
Romanovna	Rosalind	Rossalyn	Rue		Saeth
Rome	Rosalinda	Rosse	Ruel	Saadet	Safa
Romea	Rosalinde	Rosselyn	Rufa	Saar	Safara
Romia	Rosaline	Rossitza	Rufina	Saara	Safari
Romilda	Rosalyn	Rostislava	Rui	Saarah	Safeyya
Romilde	Rosalynn	Rosy	Rulza	Saasha	Saffi
Romilly	Rosamar	Rouble	Rumaysa	Saba	Saffir
Romina	Rosamaria	Rousseau	Rumba	Sabah	Saffron
Romney	Rosamond	Roux	Rumer	Sabana	Safiya
Romola	Rosamonde	Rowa	Rumi	Sabeen	Safiyah
Romy	Rosamund	Rowan	Rumina	Sabella	Safiyya
Rona	Rosana	Rowann	Rumor	Sabelle	Saga

Sagara	Salima	Sana	Sarda	Satya	Scotlyn
Sage	Salimah	Sanaa	Sardinia	Satyana	Scotlynn
Sagira	Salina	Sanam	Sarea	Satyavati	Scotty
Sagittarius	Salla	Sanaz	Sareh	Sauda	Scout
Sahalie	Salliann	Sancha	Sarelia	Saundra	Scyler
Sahar	Sallie	Sanchia	Saretha	Saura	Scylla
Sahara	Sally	Sancia	Sarff	Sausha	Sea
Saharra	Salma	Sancta	Sari	Savana	Seadhna
Sahirah	Salmon	Sandra	Sariah	Savanah	Seal
Sahkyo	Saloma	Sandrine	Sariandi	Savanna	Sean
Sahrahsahe	Salome	Sandy	Sarika	Savannah	Seana
Sahsha	Saloso	Sania	Sarina	Savara	Seanna
Sahteene	Salvadora	Saniya	Sarinna	Savarna	Searlait
Sai	Salvatora	Saniyah	Sarit	Savastian	Season
Saida	Salvia	Sanja	Sarita	Savastianova	Seath
Saidah	Salwah	Sanjeet	Sarki	Savea	Sebastiana
Saidi	Sam	Sanjita	Sarla	Saveria	Sebastiane
Saige	Samah	Sanjna	Sarni	Savina	Sebastiene
Saija	Samala	Sanna	Saroja	Saviolla	Sebbie
Sailor	Saman	Sanne	Sarra	Savita	Sebille
Saima	Samanda	Sanny	Sarrah	Savitari	Sebrina
Saint	Samanntha	Sansa	Sarriah	Savvy	Secia
Saisha	Samantha	Santa	Sarrina	Sawni	Secret
Saison	Samar	Santana	Sarva	Sawyer	Secunda
Sakaala	Samara	Santuzza	Sarya	Saxen	Seda
Sakari	Samaria	Sanura	Sasa	Saxon	Sedna
Sakhmet	Samarina	Sany	Sascha	Saxona	Sedona
Saki	Samarra	Sanya	Sasha	Saxton	Seeley
Sakina	Sambo	Sanyu	Sashah	Saya	Seelia
Sakinah	Sameh	Saoirse	Sashana	Sayaka	Seema
Saku	Sameria	Sapir	Sashenka	Sayer	Sefarina
Sakura	Sameya	Sapira	Sashi	Saylah	Sefton
Sakurako	Sami	Sapozhnika	Sashia	Saylor	Seghen
Sal	Samia	Sapphira	Sashka	Sayuri	Segovia
Sala	Samiha	Sapphire	Sashlyn	Sbyslava	Segulah
Salali	Samiira	Sappho	Sasilvia	Scarla	Segunda
Salama	Samina	Sara	Saskia	Scarlet	Seiko
Salamah	Samira	Saraa	Sassaba	Scarlett	Seina
Salamanca	Samirah	Sarabi	Sassandra	Scarlette	Seirye
Salamasina	Samirra	Sarafina	Sasson	Schantelle	Sekhet
Salana	Samiya	Sarah	Satchel	Schatzi	Sela
Salbatora	Samiyah	Sarahi	Satin	Schlomit	Selah
Saleema	Sammantha	Sarai	Satine	Scholastica	Selam
Saleena	Sammara	Saraid	Satinka	Schuyler	Selas
Salem	Sammy	Saraii	Sato	Scirocco	Selby
Salena	Samoa	Saralee	Satomi	Scoop	Seldanna
Salene	Samoset	Sarama	Satsuki	Scorpio	Sele
Salette	Sampaguita	Saran	Satu	Scota	Seleena
Saliha	Samuela	Sarane	Saturday	Scotia	Selena
Salihah	Samya	Sarayi	Saturnina	Scotland	Selene

Selenna	Serafine	Sevita	Shalona	Shara	Shawn
Selenne	Serah	Seyah	Shalonda	Sharaera	Shawna
Seleta	Seraphim	Sezja	Shalyn	Sharai	Shawnacy
Selia	Seraphina	Sfandra	Shamara	Shardae	Shawnda
Selianka	Seraphine	Shaana	Shamira	Sharde	Shawnee
Selima	Sereena	Shaaron	Shammis	Shardea	Shawnna
Selina	Serefina	Shabahang	Shan	Sharee	Shay
Selinna	Seren	Shachar	Shan-	Sharell	Shaya
Selivankov	Serena	Shada	Shana	Sharen	Shayla
Selivankova	Serenade	Shadan	Shanae	Shari	Shaylee
Selma	Serendipity	Shadell	Shanahan	Shariann	Shaylla
Selphie	Serene	Shadi	Shanda	Sharianne	Shaylynn
Selussa	Serenella	Shadiya	Shandalar	Sharifa	Shayna
Selvi	Serenity	Shadow	Shandi	Sharik	Shayne
Sema	Serenna	Shadowmoon	Shandra	Sharina	Shaynee
Semadar	Serennity	Shae	Shandy	Sharis	Shaynna
Semah	Sergia	Shaelan	Shane	Sharise	Shaynne
Semaj	Serhilda	Shafaqat	Shanee	Sharla	Shazi
Semele	Serihilda	Shafiqa	Shaneika	Sharlae	Shazzwa
Semenova	Serihilde	Shafira	Shanelle	Sharlene	Shcastna
Semenovskaia	Serilda	Shahaka	Shanese	Sharmaine	Shchastna
Semira	Serilde	Shahan	Shanessa	Sharmila	She-
Semiramis	Serissa	Shahar	Shanetha	Sharne	Shea
Semislava	Serleena	Shahira	Shani	Sharon	Sheba
Sen	Serlina	Shahla	Shania	Sharona	Shedra
Sena	Serra	Shahnaz	Shanice	Sharonda	Sheedra
Senalda	Serrena	Shaila	Shaniece	Sharonn	Sheehan
Senara	Serrenity	Shaimaa	Shaniqua	Sharpay	Sheela
Sence	Servane	Shaina	Shaniya	Sharri	Sheelah
Seneca	Serwa	Shaindel	Shanley	Sharron	Sheena
Senegal	Sesame	Shaine	Shanna	Sharvani	Sheenna
Senga	Sesen	Shainna	Shannae	Shasa	Sheera
Senia	Sesheta	Shaked	Shannan	Shasha	Sheherazade
Senna	Sessilee	Shakeela	Shannee	Shashi	Sheherezade
Senny	Seth	Shakila	Shannen	Shasta	Sheila
Senona	Sethe	Shakina	Shannia	Shasti	Sheiletta
Senorita	Setia	Shakira	Shannon	Shateque	Sheilla
Senta	Setsuko	Shakirah	Shanonn	Shatoya	Shel
Seosaimhthin	Sevan	Shakti	Shanta	Shaula	Shelagh
Sephora	Sevastianiia	Shalan	Shantal	Shauna	Shelah
September	Sevastiiana	Shalana	Shantell	Shaundra	Shelbe
Septima	Sevda	Shalendra	Shantelle	Shaunna	Shelbee
Sequence	Seven	Shalheira	Shanti	Shaunta	Shelbey
Sequester	Severin	Shalhevet	Shanton	Shavonn	Shelbi
Sequin	Severina	Shalimar	Shany	Shavonne	Shelbie
Sequoia	Severine	Shalin	Shanyrria	Shavsha	Shelby
Sequoyah	Sevgi	Shalini	Shaquana	Shaw	Sheldon
Sera	Sevigne	Shalisa	Shaquanna	Shawanna	Shelee
Serafima	Sevilen	Shalom	Shaquilla	Shawano	Shelette
Serafina	Sevilla	Shalon	Shaquitta	Shawdi	Shell

112

Shellbie	Shinobu	Sibeal	Simcha	Siuiunbek	Sneha
Shellby	Shiori	Sibila	Simeona	Siuiunbeka	Snejana
Shelley	Shira	Sibley	Simi	Siuiunbuka	Snigurka
Shellie	Shiran	Sibyl	Simin	Siunbek	Snow
Shelly	Shiraz	Sibyla	Simla	Siunbeka	Snowdrop
Shelovlevaya	Shiri	Sibylla	Simmone	Siusan	SnowFlower
Shemeka	Shiriaeva	Sicily	Simona	Siv	SnowWhite
Shena	Shirin	Sidda	Simone	Sivan	Snowy
Shenandoah	Shirina	Siddalee	Simonetta	Sive	Sobina
Shenna	Shirkia	Sidera	Simonne	Sivney	Socorra
Shepry	Shirlene	Sidney	Simplicity	Sixsipita	Socorro
Shera	Shirley	Sidone	Simra	Sixtine	Sofeia
Sherene	Shirlyn	Sidonia	Sina	Siyanda	Soffia
Sheri	Shiva	Sidonie	Sinasta	Siyona	Sofi
Sheridan	Shivani	Sidony	Sincere	Skameikina	Sofia
Sherie	Shizuka	Sidorova	Sincerely	Skanawati	Sofie
Sherilyn	Shizuko	Sidra	Sincerity	Skate	Sofieke
Sherine	Shkonka	Siegfrieda	Sinclair	Skena	Sofiia
Sherisa	Shlomit	Siena	Sine	Skky	Sofiya
Sherise	Shobha	Sienna	Sinead	Skonka	Sohalia
Sherleen	Shobi	Sierra	Sineaid	Skule	Sojourner
Sherley	Shomecossee	Sigal	Sineidin	Sky	Sokanon
Sherlyn	Shona	Sigalit	Sinklitikiia	Skye	Soki
Sherrerd	Shoneah	Sigfreda	Sinnafain	Skyee	Sokw
Sherri	Shoney	Sigismonda	Sinopa	Skyla	Sol
Sherridan	Shoshana	Signa	Sintra	Skylaa	Sola
Sherrill	Shoshanah	Signe	Siny	Skylaar	Solada
Sherry	Shoshanna	Signilda	Siobahn	Skylar	Solaina
Sherryll	Shoshone	Signy	Siobhán	Skylarr	Solaine
Sheryl	Shoushan	Sigourney	Siofra	Skyler	Solana
Sheryll	Shreya	Sigrid	Siona	Skylla	Solange
Shesheba	Shuang	Sigun	Sioned	Skyllar	Solara
Sheshebens	ShuFang	Sigune	Siouxsie	Skyye	Solaris
Shevaughn	Shui	Sihu	Sira	Slaine	Soledad
Shevonne	Shukriya	Sika	Siran	Slainie	Soledada
Sheyla	Shula	Silana	Sirena	Slania	Soleil
Sheylla	Shulamit	Sile	Siri	Slanie	Solene
Shia	Shulamith	Sileas	Siria	Slany	Soliania
Shialacvar	Shuman	Silence	Siriol	Slate	Solita
Shiela	Shun	Sileny	Sirvat	Slava	Solon
Shields	Shura	Silja	Sisika	Slavna	Solona
Shierlyn	Shushanika	Silke	Sisley	Sloan	Solone
Shifra	Shvakova	Silken	Sissela	Sloane	Solstice
Shila	Shyael	Silvana	Sissy	Smadar	Solveig
Shiloah	Shyann	Silver	Sistine	Smilla	Solymar
Shiloh	Shyanne	Silvestra	Sitala	Smils	Soma
Shima	Shyla	Silvia	Sitanka	Smina	Somatra
Shimona	Shylla	Silvine	Sitara	Smirenka	Somer
Shimrit	Sian	Sima	Sitembileq	Snana	Somers
Shinju	Siany	Simbala	Sitka	Snanduliia	Sommer

Sona	Sparrow	Stefannie	Suchin	Susane	Sweeney
Sonata	Spasenieva	Stefanova	Sudehna	Susann	Swoosie
Sonatina	Spencer	Stefanya	Sudekhna	Susanna	Sy
Sonaya	Spera	Steffani	Sudila	Susannah	Sy'Rai
Sondra	Speranza	Steffanie	Sue	Susanne	Sybella
Sonechka	Spes	Steffi	Sueanne	Sushi	Sybil
Sonel	Spirit	Steffie	Suelita	Susie	Sybylla
Sonia	Spitoslava	Stella	Suellen	Susklahava	Sydelle
Sonja	Spitsislava	Stellan	Suewinda	Susmita	Sydnee
Sonnagh	Sprig	Steltella	Sufa	Suspiria	Sydney
Sonnehilda	Spring	Stepanida	Sugar	Sussan	Sydni
Sonnet	Springer	Stepanova	Suhana	Sussie	Sydnie
Sonnia	Spruce	Stephaine	Sukey	Sutherland	Syesha
Sonnya	Squire	Stephana	Suki	Sutton	Syler
Sonoma	Stacci	Stephania	Sula	Suvi	Syllis
Sonomi	Stacey	Stephanie	Sulislava	Suzan	Sylmae
Sonora	Stacia	Stephany	Sullivan	Suzanna	Sylvana
Sonya	Stacie	Stepka	Sully	Suzannah	Sylvia
Sonyuru	Stacy	Sterling	Sulola	Suzanne	Sylvie
Sonyusha	Stam	Sterre	Sultana	Suzelly	Sylwia
Sonyushka	Stamatina	Stesha	Sulwyn	Suzetta	Symber
Sookie	Stana	Stetson	Suma	Suzette	Symislava
Sooleawa	Stanislava	Stevany	Sumana	Suzu	Symona
Soora	Stanka	Steveanna	Sumaya	Suzuki	Symphony
Sophelia	Stanley	Stevie	Sumayah	Suzume	Symrustar
Sophi	Stansie	Stevonna	Sumer	Suzy	Syndra
Sophia	Star	Stina	Sumi	Svakhna	Synnove
Sophie	Starbuck	Stockard	Sumiko	Svana	Syona
Sophiee	Starla	Stolma	Sumitra	Svante	Syp
Sophronia	Starleen	Stolpolcha	Summer	Svara	Sypovaia
Sora	Starley	Stopolcha	Sumorokova	Svatata	Syreeta
Soraya	Starlin	Storm	Sun	Svatava	Syrita
Sorcha	Starling	Stormi	Suna	Svatochna	Syshe
Sorena	Starlyn	Stormie	Sundari	Svatohna	Syviis
Sorina	Starr	Stormin	Sunday	Svea	
Soroka	Starrla	Stormy	Sundown	Sveisla	**T**
Sorrel	Starsha	Story	Sunee	Sveta	
Sorrell	Stasia	Stranizlava	Sunila	Svetlana	Taana
Sorsasta	Stasy	Stratka	Sunita	Svetocha	Taara
Sosanna	Stasya	Strawberry	Sunki	Svetokhna	Tabananica
Sosfena	Stav	Strezhena	Sunklitikiia	Sviatata	Tabassum
Sosi	Steel	Strezhislava	Sunniva	Sviatokhna	Tabatha
Sosie	Steena	Strezislava	Sunny	Sviatoslava	Tabbatha
Sosipatra	Steevie	Struan	Sunshine	Svoda	Tabbetha
Sotsona	Stefani	Struana	Suri	Swaantje	Tabbitha
Soubrette	Stefania	Stylanie	Suria	Swachnina	Tabby
Southern	Stefanida	Suave	Suruchi	Swanhild	Tabetha
Sovann	Stefanidka	Subhan	Surya	Swann	Tabia
Soyala	Stefanie	Subira	Susan	Swatawa	Tabina
Sparkle	Stefanni	Suchi	Susana	Sweden	Tabitha

Tablita	Tainn	Talori	Tamiya	Tanisha	Tarren
Tabor	Taipa	Talula	Tamma	Tanita	Tarsha
Tabora	Taisce	Talulah	Tammara	Tanith	Taruh
Taborri	Taisha	Talulla	Tammarra	Taniya	Taryn
Tacey	Taishineia	Talullah	Tammeka	Taniyah	Tarynn
Tacha	Taisie	Talya	Tammera	Tanja	Tasanee
Tachia	Taisiia	Tam	Tammi	Tanka	Tasenka
Tachiana	Taisiya	Tama	Tammia	Tankaku	Tash
Tachianna	Tait	Tamah	Tammie	Tanna	Tasha
Taci	Taite	Tamako	Tammika	Tannar	Tashana
Tacincala	Taj	Tamal	Tammra	Tanner	Tasheika
Tacita	Taja	Tamala	Tammy	Tannia	Tashia
Tacy	Takako	Tamami	Tamora	Tannika	Tashiana
Tadewi	Takala	Taman	Tamra	Tannis	Tashianna
Tadi	Takara	Tamanna	Tamryn	Tannisha	Tashina
Tadita	Takoda	Tamar	Tamsin	Tanniya	Tashira
Taelar	Tal	Tamara	Tamsyn	Tannya	Tashiya
Taeler	Tala	Tamarah	Tamyra	Tansy	Tasia
Taelor	Talaith	Tamarice	Tana	Tanuja	Tasmin
Taenya	Talanashta	Tamarind	Tanaa	Tanwen	Tasmine
Tafariah	Talar	Tamarisk	Tanalia	Tanya	Tasnim
Taffeta	Talasi	Tamarix	Tanaquil	Tao	Tassa
Taffy	Talayeh	Tamarr	Tanasha	Tapa	Tassia
Tahigwa	Talbot	Tamarra	Tanaya	Tapanga	Tassie
Tahira	Tale	Tamary	Tancy	Tappen	Tasunke
Tahirah	Tali	Tamasha	Tandice	Tara	Tasya
Tahiti	Talia	Tamasine	Tandra	Taraann	Tata
Tahiya	Taliah	Tamatha	Tandula	Tarachand	Tate
Tahki	Talicia	Tamayo	Tandy	Taraja	Tatelyn
Tahlia	Taliesin	Tambe	Tanea	Taraji	Tati
Tahn	Talila	Tamber	Tanechka	Tarala	Tatiana
Tahna	Talindra	Tambika	Taneisha	Tarana	Tatianka
Tahnee	Taline	Tambra	Tanesha	Tarangini	Tatianna
Tahnia	Talisa	Tameeka	Tanessa	Tarannum	Tatiiana
Tahniya	Talise	Tameera	Taneya	Tarasynora	Tatjana
Tahnya	Talisha	Tameka	Tanga	Tarbula	Tatsa
Tahoe	Talissa	Tamekka	Tangela	Taree	Tattiana
Tahsha	Talitha	Tamera	Tangerine	Taregan	Tattianna
Tai	Taliyah	Tamerlane	Tangia	Tarhe	Tattyana
Taidula	Talleen	Tamerra	Tangie	Tari	Tatum
Taifa	Talli	Tamesis	Tangier	Tarian	Tatyana
Taigi	Tallia	Tami	Tanginika	Tariana	Tatyanna
Taika	Tallie	Tamia	Tangwen	Tarika	Taunia
Tailer	Tallis	Tamiia	Tani	Tarin	Taunya
Tailor	Tallulah	Tamiika	Tania	Tarisai	Taura
Tailynn	Tally	Tamika	Taniel	Tarleton	Tauret
Taima	Tallys	Tamikka	Tanija	Tarlo	Tauri
Taimi	Talma	Tamiko	Tanika	Tarot	Tauria
Taina	Talor	Tamira	Tanikka	Tarra	Taurus
Taini	Talora	Tamitha	Tanis	Tarragon	Tava

115

Tavaril	Teala	Tempo	Terry	Thasha	Thu
Tavi	Teamhair	Tendai	Terryal	Thasitalia	Thuong
Tavia	Teangi	Tender	Terryl	Thea	Thuraia
Tavianna	Teasagh	Tene	Tertia	Theanna	Thuraya
Tavita	Teasha	Teneil	Teryani	Thecla	Thurayya
Tavlunbeka	Techiya	Teness	Teryl	Theda	Thurl
Tavora	Tecla	Tenisha	Terza	Theia	Thuy
Tawana	Tecumseh	Tenley	Tesheia	Thekla	Thwayya
Tawnee	Teddi	Tennessee	Teshi	Thelma	Thy
Tawney	Tedra	Tenoch	Teshka	Thelonius	Thyme
Tawni	Teea	Tenskwatawa	Tesia	Thelred	Thyra
Tawnia	Teela	Tenzin	Tesla	Thema	Tia
Tawnie	Teenie	Teodora	Tess	Themba	Tiaa
Tawny	Tefnut	Teodory	Tessa	Themis	Tiaga
Tawnya	Tegan	Teodozji	Tessica	Thenjiwe	Tiahna
Taworri	Tegeen	Teofila	Tessie	Theo	Tiana
Tay	Tegwen	Tequila	Tetka	Theodora	Tianna
Taya	Teha	Tequilla	Tetsu	Theodorsia	Tiara
Tayana	Teharissa	Tera	Tetty	Theodosia	Tiaret
Tayanita	Tehila	Terah	Teva	Theola	Tiarra
Tayden	Tehya	Teranika	Tevin	Theone	Tiassale
Taye	Teige	Terceira	Tevkel	Theophaneia	Tiatha
Tayen	Teigra	Terehasa	Tevy	Theophania	Tiauna
Tayla	Teila	Terema	Tex	Theophila	Tibbie
Taylah	Teisha	Terena	Texana	Theophilia	Tibby
Taylar	Teja	Terencia	Texas	Theora	Tiberia
Taylee	Tejana	Terentia	Teya	Thera	Tibone
Tayler	Tekh	Teresa	Teyemthohisa	Theresa	Tieesha
Taylin	Tekha	Teresia	Teyla	Therese	Tien
Tayllor	Tekla	Teresina	Teylor	Theresia	Tiernan
Taylor	Tekli	Teresita	Tferianka	Theressa	Tierney
Taylore	Tekusa	Teressa	Thackary	Theria	Tierra
Taylour	Telema	Teretha	Thaddea	Therma	Tiesha
Taylre	Teleri	Tereza	Thadina	Theron	Tieve
Tayna	Teles	Teri	Thadine	Thessaly	Tifany
Taysia	Telissa	Teriann	Thady	Theta	Tifara
Taysir	Telma	Terilynn	Thaimy	Thetis	Tiferet
Tayte	Telsa	Terpsichore	Thais	Thi	Tiffani
Tayten	Telyn	Terra	Thaïs	Thina	Tiffanii
Tazanna	Tema	Terrah	Thalassa	Thirza	Tiffanie
Tazara	Teme	Terran	Thalia	Thisbe	Tiffany
Tazia	Temima	Terrene	Thames	Thomae	Tiffney
Tazu	Temina	Terresa	Thamina	Thomasa	Tiger
Tchondee	Temira	Terressa	Thana	Thomasin	Tigernach
Téa	Tempe	Terri	Thandie	Thomasina	Tigris
Teagan	Temperance	Terrian	Thandiwe	Thomsina	Tiina
Teagann	Tempest	Terrica	Thane	Thono	Tijuana
Teagin	Tempeste	Terrie	Thanh	Thora	Tikva
Teah	Templa	Terris	Thao	Thornleigh	Tikvah
Teal	Temple	Terrwyn	Thaola	Thornlie	Tilda

Tilde	Tiuu	Tonicia	Totsi	Trinh	Tsukiko
Tille	Tiva	Tonii	Tottie	Trini	Tsungani
Tillie	Tivian	Tonja	Totty	Trinidad	Tsvetanka
Tilly	Tivka	Tonni	Toula	Trinitty	Tsvetkova
Tiltilla	Tivona	Tonnia	Tourmaline	Trinity	Tu
Timandra	Tiwesdaeg	Tonniya	Tova	Trinna	Tuesday
Timber	Tiya	Tonnya	Tovah	Trinnity	Tugenda
Timberly	Tiyana	Tony	Tove	Trish	Tula
Timea	Tiyanna	Tonya	Tovi	Trisha	Tulia
Timi	Tkalis	Topanga	Toya	Trishna	Tuliana
Timia	Tlalli	Topaz	Toyah	Triska	Tulip
Timila	Tmira	Topper	Trace	Trista	Tullia
Timothea	Toan	Topsy	Tracen	Tristabelle	Tully
Timothia	Toba	Tora	Tracey	Tristan	Tulna
Tina	Tobi	Toral	Traci	Tristana	Tulsa
Tinble	Tobin	Torberta	Traciella	Tristann	Tulsi
Tindra	Tobit	Tordis	Tracy	Tristany	Tumaini
Ting	Toby	Toree	Trakiala	Tristessa	Tunder
Tinley	Toccara	Toreth	Tram	Tristina	Tundra
Tinna	Toccata	Torey	Trang	Tristyn	Tupelo
Tinsley	Tochtli	Tori	Tranquilina	Triveni	Turia
Tiombe	Todorka	Toria	Tranquility	Trixi	Turkessa
Tiona	Toibe	Toriana	Tranquilla	Trixie	Turquoise
Tionna	Toinette	Torie	Trapper	Trixy	Tutana
Tip	Toireasa	Toril	Traveler	Troian	Tuulia
Tiphanie	Toki	Torille	Traviata	Troika	Tuva
Tiponi	Tokori	Torilyn	Trea	Tropica	Tuwa
Tiponya	Tokyo	Torlan	Treasa	Troya	Tuyen
Tipper	Tolinka	Tornado	Treasure	Trpena	Tuyet
Tippi	Tolla	Torokanova	Treat	Truda	Tvisha
Tira	Toltecatl	Torra	Treena	Trude	Tvoislava
Tiriara	Toma	Torrance	Treise	Trudie	Tvoyzlava
Tirion	Tomai	Torree	Trelane	Trudy	Tvuna
Tiryns	Tomasina	Torrell	Trella	Trufena	Twain
Tirza	Tomasine	Torrey	Tress	Trula	Twila
Tirzah	Tomi	Torri	Tressa	Truly	Twilight
Tis-see-woo-na-tis	Tomiko	Torrie	Treszka	Truma	Twyla
	Tomila	Torrin	Tretiakovskaia	Trung	Ty
Tisa	Tomislava	Tory	Treva	Trusha	Tyanne
Tish	Tomoe	Tosca	Trevon	Truth	Tyas
Tisha	Tomoka	Toseland	Triage	Tryna	Tycen
Tisharu	Tomoko	Tosha	Trianna	Tryphena	Tyipa
Tishka	Tomomi	Toshawah	Tribeca	Tsaritsa	Tykaja
Tishkina	Tomoyo	Toshi	Tricia	Tsarra	Tyler
Tita	Tonasha	Toshiana	Trilby	Tsifira	Tylie
Titania	Tonaya	Toshie	Trillare	Tsila	Tyme
Titian	Tonechka	Tosia	Trillian	Tsiyone	Tymeria
Titiana	Toni	Tossa	Trina	Tsubaki	Tynan
Titka	Tonie	Totie	Trinetta	Tsubame	Tyne
Tiutcheva	Tonia	Totole	Trinette	Tsubasa	Tynice

117

Tyra	Ulf	Urania	Valarie	Vanja	Vasundhara
Tyran	Ulfah	Urbain	Valda	Vanmra	Vasya
Tyree	Uli	Urban	Valdis	Vanna	Vatusia
Tyrique	Ulia	Urbana	Vale	Vannesa	Vaughn
Tyro	Uliaanitsa	Urbi	Valechka	Vannessa	Vaviia
Tyronica	Uliana	Uri	Valen	Vannah	Vea
Tyrra	Ulianiia	Uriana	Valencia	Vanora	Veanna
Tysheenia	Ulianka	Urice	Valene	Vanya	Veata
Tyson	Ulianushka	Uriela	Valenta	Vara	Vecepia
Tytti	Uliasha	Urit	Valentina	Varali	Veda
Tyyne	Ulicia	Urja	Valentine	Varana	Vedetta
Tzadika	Uliiana	Urmi	Valentinna	Varda	Vedette
Tzefira	Ulima	Urmicca	Valera	Vardit	Vedia
Tzeitel	Ulita	Ursa	Valeraine	Vared	Veera
Tzigane	Ull	Ursala	Valere	Varenka	Veerle
Tzila	Ulla	Urshila	Valeria	Variel	Vega
Tzilla	Ulrica	Ursula	Valerie	Varina	Vegas
Tziona	Ulrika	Ursulina	Valeska	Varinia	Vela
Tzipora	Ulrike	Ursulla	Valetta	Varinka	Velatha
Tziporah	Ulrikee	Urvi	Vali	Varka	Velda
Tzippa	Ultima	Uschymna	Valiant	Varsha	Velia
Tzipporah	Ulu	Usha	Valindra	Varsonofia	Velika
Tzirel	Ululani	Usoa	Valkyrie	Vartoughi	Velislava
Tzivia	Ulva	Usra	Valle	Vartouhi	Vella
Tzivya	Ulyana	Ustenia	Vallerie	Vartsislava	Velma
Tziyona	Ulyciana	Ustiniia	Valley	Varushka	Velouté
Tzofia	Ulyssa	Uta	Vallombrosa	Varvara	Velvet
Tzuriya	Ulyssia	Utah	Valmai	Varya	Venda
Tzzipporah	Uma	Utari	Valo	Varyusha	Vendela
	Umatilla	Uttara	Valonia	Vasant	Venecia
	Umay	Uvatera	Valor	Vasanta	Venerada
U	Umaymah	Uyen	Valora	Vasanti	Venessa
	Ume	Uzima	Valorie	Vasha	Venetia
Uaine	Umeko	Uzma	Valterra	Vashti	Venezia
Ualda	Umi	Uzuri	Valtina	Vasileva	Venice
Ualentina	Umika	Uzziye	Valya	Vasilevna	Ventana
Uatchit	Umm		Van	Vasilevskaia	Ventseslava
Uberta	Ummi	**V**	Vanda	Vasilia	Ventura
Udele	Umnia		Vandana	Vasilida	Venus
Ugur	Umut	Vada	Vanesa	Vasilievaia	Venya
Uheri	Una	Vadit	Vanessa	Vasilii	Vera
Uirko	Undine	Vaetild	Vanetta	Vasiliki	Veradisia
Ujana	Unefiia	Vafara	Vangie	Vasilina	Verbena
Ula	Unique	Vahn	Vanhi	Vasilisa	Verbenia
Ulalia	Unity	Vail	Vania	Vasilissa	Verda
Ulan	Unka	Vakhneva	Vanida	Vasilista	Verdad
Ulana	Unna	Vakhtina	Vanig	Vasisa	Verde
Ulani	Uny	Val	Vanille	Vassa	Verdi
Uleia	Upritsa	Vala	Vanita	Vassillissa	Vered
Ulelesse	Ura		Vanity	Vasudha	Verena
Ulen'ka					

118

Verina	Vickki	Vinnie	Vivienne	Vulpine	Waseemah
Verity	Vicky	Viola	Viviette	Vyesna	Washakie
Verlee	Victoire	Violante	Vivka	Vyomini	Wasila
Verlene	Victoria	Violet	Vlada	Vyra	Watchemonne
Vermilion	Victoriana	Violett	Vladaia	Vysheslava	Waterfall
Vermont	Victorina	Violetta	Vladilena	Vyshia	Wattan
Verna	Victorine	Violette	Vladilenaova		Wauna
Vernon	Victorria	Viollette	Vladimira	**W**	Wava
Verochka	Vicuska	Vionaika	Vladisava		Waverly
Verona	Vida	Vione	Vladislava	Waapalaa	Wavery
Veronica	Vidette	Vionnet	Vladka	Wabanang	Wawa
Veronika	Vidonia	Viradecthis	Vladlena	Wade	Wawinges
Veronikeia	Vieira	Virag	Vlaikha	Wafa	Waynette
Veronique	Vienna	Virdia	Vlastika	Wafiya	Waynoka
Veronnica	Viera	Virendra	Vlcena	Waheeda	Wealote
Verrona	Vigdis	Virgilia	Vlora	Wahmenitu	Wednesday
Verronica	Vigee	Virginee	Vlschet	Wahponjea	Wei
Verronique	Vigilia	Virginia	Vogna	Wakana	Welcome
Vershina	Vignetta	Virginnia	Voina	Wakanda	Welislawa
Veruca	Vignette	Virgo	Voislava	Wakapa	Wellesley
Veruschka	Viheke	Viridiana	Volante	Wakaun	Wellington
Vervain	Viivi	Virika	Voleta	Wakechai	Welmoed
Verve	Vika	Virineia	Voletta	Waki	Wen
Vesna	Vikashenka	Vironikiia	Volodimerna	Wakinyela	Wenda
Vesper	Vikki	Virtue	Volotka	Walburga	Wendelin
Vespera	Viktoria	Visala	Volotkoveia	Walda	Wendell
Vesta	Viktorie	Vishemila	Volotok	Waldhurga	Wendelle
Vestele	Viktoriya	Visitacion	Volusia	Waldina	Wendi
Veta	Vila	Visola	Volva	Waleska	Wendie
Vetenega	Vilayna	Vita	Von	Walidah	Wendy
Vevay	Vilda	Vitalia	Vonda	Walker	Wenndy
Veveia	Vilena	Vitalya	Vondila	Walkiria	Wenona
Vevila	Vilenina	Vitasa	Vondra	Wallace	Wenopa
Vevina	Vilhelmina	Vitko	Vonte	Wallis	Weronikia
Vi	Vilina	Vitla	Vor	Walta	Weshcubb
Via	Ville	Vitoslava	Voshell	Waltrina	Weslan
Viachenega	Villetta	Vittoria	Voss	Walvia	Weslee
Vian	Villette	Viva	Vova	Wan	Wesley
Vianca	Vilma	Viveca	Vox	Wanda	Weslyn
Vianna	Vilna	Viveka	Voyzlava	Wande	West
Vianne	Vimala	Vivi	Vrai	Wandella	Westley
Vianne	Vina	Vivia	Vrata	Waneta	Westlyn
Viansola	Vinanti	Vivian	Vratislava	Wanetta	Whaley
Viatrix	Vinata	Viviana	Vrkhuslava	Wangari	Whimsy
Vic	Vinaya	Viviane	Vrotsislava	Wannon	Whisper
Vica	Vincentia	Viviann	Vrsanka	Wanyecha	Whit
Vice	Vine	Vivianna	Vseslava	Warda	Whitley
Vicenta	Vinga	Vivianne	Vui	Wardah	Whitnee
Vicenza	Vinia	Vivica	Vukosava	Warna	Whitney
Vickii	Vinita	Vivien	Vukoslava	Warvara	Whitni

Whitnie	Winifred	Wynter	Ximenia	Yakira	Yashira
Whittley	Winka	Wyome	Ximenna	Yalanilue	Yasiman
Whittney	Winnie	Wyoming	Xin	Yale	Yasma
Whizdom	Winnifred	Wysandra	Xinavane	Yalena	Yasmeen
Whoopi	Winnona		Xing	Yalenchka	Yasmeena
Wibeke	Winola	**X**	XingXing	Yalens	Yasmen
Wicahpi	Winona		XinQian	Yaletha	Yasmiin
Wicapiwakan	Winslet	Xabrina	Xio	Yalgonata	Yasmin
Widad	Winslow	Xalbadora	Xiomara	Yalitza	Yasmina
Wiebke	Winsome	Xalvadora	Xiomarys	Yamha	Yasmine
Wierga	Winta	Xanadu	Xipil	Yamilet	Yassah
Wies	Winter	Xandra	Xiu	Yamileth	Yassmin
Wiesje	Winterlynn	Xandy	Xiuhcoatl	Yamin	Yassmine
Wihakayda	Wira	Xannon	XiuJuan	Yamina	Yasu
Wihe	Wirke	Xantara	Xochitl	Yaminah	Yates
Wikimak	Wisconsin	Xanthe	Xois	Yamka	Yathlanae
Wikitoria	Wisdom	Xanthene	Xola	Yamparti	Yatima
Wikolia	Wish	Xanthia	Xolani	Yan	Yauvani
Wikta	Wissa	Xanthipe	Xuan	Yana	Yavesly
Wiktorja	Wistar	Xanthippe	Xue	Yanamaria	Yaxha
Wilda	Wisteria	Xantho	XueFang	Yanamarie	Yazmin
Wileen	Witoslava	Xanti	Xuxa	Yancey	Yazzmin
Wiley	Wiwka	Xaria	Xyla	Yancy	Ydel
Wilfreda	Wladyka	Xarissa	Xyleena	Yaneisy	Yeardleigh
Wilhelma	Woape	Xava	Xylia	Yanely	Yeardley
Wilhelmina	Woina	Xaviera	Xyliana	Yanenowi	Yeats
Wilhelmine	Woksapiwi	Xaviere	Xylina	Yanichel	Yedid
Wilhemina	Wowashi	Xavierra	Xylona	Yanire	Yedida
Will	Wozhupiwi	Xavierre		Yank	Yedidah
Willa	Wrata	Xen	**Y**	Yanka	Yehudit
Willamena	Wratislava	Xena		Yankee	Yekaterina
Willemijn	Wren	Xeni	Yaakova	Yannick	Yelena
Willemina	Wrocislawa	Xenia	Yaakove	Yantse	Yelina
Willene	Wuti	Xenna	Yaasmeen	Yaotl	Yelisabeta
Willette	Wyanet	Xenobia	Yachi	Yapany	Yelizavetam
Williamina	Wyeth	Xenophon	Yachne	Yara	Yelysaveta
Willma	Wyetta	Xeraphina	Yadira	Yardena	Yemena
Willow	Wylda	Xevera	Yadra	Yardenah	Yenge
Wilma	Wylie	Xeveria	Yael	Yardley	Yenta
Wilmet	Wyn	Xexilia	Yaereene	Yareli	Yentl
Wilmot	Wynda	Xhosa	Yafa	Yarelli	Yepa
Wilona	Wynell	Xi-wang	Yaffa	Yaretzi	Yeraldina
Wilone	Wynfreda	Xia	Yaffit	Yarina	Yerusha
Win	Wynifred	XiaHe	Yagmur	Yaritza	Yesenia
Wind	Wynn	Xiamara	Yahaira	Yarkona	Yesennia
Winda	Wynne	Xiang	Yahaloma	Yarmilla	Yessenia
Windsor	Wynnifred	XiaoChen	Yaineris	Yarona	Yessica
Windy	Wynona	XiaoHong	Yaira	Yarrow	Yetsye
Winema	Wynonna	Xidorn	Yaiza	Yas	Yetta
Wing	Wynstelle	Ximena	Yajaira	Yasemin	Yettie

Yetty	Yonina	Yukiko	Zahar	Zanobia	Zdislava
Yeva	Yoninah	Yukino	Zahara	Zanta	Zdzislaba
Yevdokiya	Yonit	Yule	Zahari	Zanthe	Zea
Yevfrosinya	Yonita	Yulenka	Zaharra	Zaphara	Zeal
Yevgeniya	Yoomee	Yulia	Zahava	Zapopa	Zealand
Yevgenya	Yordan	Yuliana	Zahavah	Zara	Zebina
Yevtsye	Yordana	Yulianiya	Zahina	Zarah	Zeborah
Yevunye	Yori	Yulika	Zahira	Zarahlinda	Zee
Ygeme	Yoruba	Yuliy	Zahra	Zarela	Zeena
Ygrainne	Yosdalkis	Yuliya	Zahrah	Zaria	Zefira
Ygritte	Yoseba	Yulmanda	Zaida	Zariah	Zefjm
Yi	Yosebe	Yulya	Zaide	Zariel	Zehava
Yifat	Yosefa	Yuma	Zaidee	Zarifa	Zehave
Yihana	Yoselin	Yumaris	Zaiden	Zarina	Zehavi
Yildiz	Yosepha	Yumi	Zaila	Zarita	Zehavit
Yimeyam	Yosephina	Yumie	Zaina	Zaritsa	Zehira
YiMin	Yoshe	Yumiko	Zainab	Zariyah	Zehuva
Yisraela	Yoshi	Yumna	Zainabu	Zariza	Zeila
Yitta	Yoshiko	Yuna	Zaira	Zarola	Zela
YiZe	Yoshino	Yuricema	Zaire	Zarouhi	Zelah
Yizel	Yoslene	Yuridia	Zajac	Zarra	Zelda
Ylva	Youko	Yuridiana	Zakharia	Zarrah	Zelena
Ynes	Youta	Yuriko	Zakharieva	Zarria	Zelene
Ynez	Yovanka	Yusmara	Zakharina	Zarya	Zelenia
Yngvild	Yovela	Yusra	Zakia	Zasha	Zelenka
Ynshael	Yoyko	Yuta	Zakiya	Zathura	Zelia
Yo	Yrlissa	Yuuna	Zakuro	Zavidovicha	Zelie
Yoad	Yrneha	Yuzuki	Zala	Zaviera	Zelig
Yoana	Yrthraethra	Yvaine	Zale	Zavorokhina	Zelina
Yocheved	Ysabel	Yvette	Zalika	Zavrina	Zelkova
Yocheved	Ysabell	Yvian	Zaliki	Zayd	Zella
Yoconda	Ysabelle	Yvonna	Zaltana	Zayda	Zelma
Yogenya	Ysanne	Yvonne	Zambda	Zayit	Zelozelos
Yogi	Ysbail		Zambezi	Zaylee	Zemira
Yohance	Yseult	**Z**	Zamiatina	Zayley	Zemirah
Yoki	Ysmyrlda		Zamora	Zaylie	Zemora
Yoko	Yu	Zaara	Zàn	Zayn	Zemorah
Yoland	Yua	Zabana	Zana	Zayna	Zen
Yolanda	Yudelle	Zabby	Zanaa	Zaynab	Zena
Yolanda-Abigail	Yudit	Zabel	Zandeleigh	Zaynah	Zenaida
	Yudita	Zabela	Zandophen	Zaza	Zenaide
Yolande	Yue	Zabelle	Zandra	Zazu	Zenas
Yolanthe	YueYan	Zabrina	Zane	Zbina	Zenaveve
Yollanda	Yuhudit	Zacharee	Zaneta	Zbinka	Zenda
Yolonda	Yui	Zada	Zanetta	Zbiska	Zendaya
Yolotli	Yuina	Zadie	Zaniah	Zbynek	Zene
Yomaira	YuJie	Zafira	Zanita	Zbynko	Zenechka
Yona	Yuka	Zafirah	Zaniyah	Zbyshka	Zenevieva
Yonah	Yukari	Zagiri	Zanna	Zdena	Zenia
Yonaidys	Yuki	Zagora	Zanns	Zdeslava	Zenith

121

Zenja	Zillah	Zofia	Zumac
Zenna	Zilpah	Zofie	Zuna
Zenobia	Zilpha	Zohara	Zuni
Zenochka	Zilya	Zohartze	Zureidy
Zenon	Zima	Zoheret	Zuri
Zeny	Zimra	Zohra	Zuria
Zenya	Zina	Zoia	Zurie
Zephan	Zinaida	Zoie	Zuriel
Zephira	Zinerva	Zoika	Zurina
Zephne	Zinna	Zoila	Zurine
Zephrine	Zinnia	Zola	Zusa
Zephyr	Zinovia	Zolynn	Zuwena
Zephyra	Zinoviia	Zona	Zuzana
Zephyrine	Zion	Zondra	Zuzanna
Zeppelin	Ziona	Zonne	Zuzanny
Zera	Zippora	Zonta	Zuzela
Zerelda	Zipporah	Zooeey	Zuzi
Zerlina	Ziraili	Zooey	Zuzu
Zerlinda	Zisel	Zora	Zvatata
Zeta	Zisse	Zorah	Zvenislava
Zetta	Zissi	Zoraida	Zvezda
Zeuxippe	Zita	Zorana	Zweena
Zeva	Zitkaduta	Zoraya	Zwi
Zevida	Zitkala	Zorea	Zyanya
Zezilia	Zitkalasa	Zorina	Zylina
Zhaleh	Zitomira	Zosia	Zyphire
Zhane	Ziv	Zosma	Zyta
Zhanna	Ziva	Zoya	Zytka
Zhdana	Zivah	Zoyenka	
Zhen	Zivanka	Zsa	
Zhena	Ziven	ZsaZsa	
Zhenga	Zixi	Zsazsa	
Zhenya	Ziya	Zsófia	
Zhi	Ziza	Zsoka	
Zhirava	Zizi	Zsuska	
Zhivana	Zlata	Ztrezena	
Zhona	Zlhna	Zubaida	
Zhonka	Znata	Zubeda	
Zi	Zo	Zudora	
Zia	Zoan	Zuelia	
Ziarre	Zoanne	Zula	
Ziazan	Zoastria	Zuleika	
Zibby	Zocha	Zuleikha	
Zibia	Zody	Zulema	
Zibiah	Zoe	Zulie	
Zigana	Zoee	Zulima	
Zihna	Zoeey	Zulimar	
Zila	Zoelle	Zulma	
Zilke	Zoey	Zuly	
Zilla	Zofeia	Zuma	

Printed in Great Britain
by Amazon.co.uk, Ltd.,
Marston Gate.